With**CHILD**

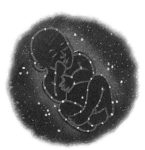

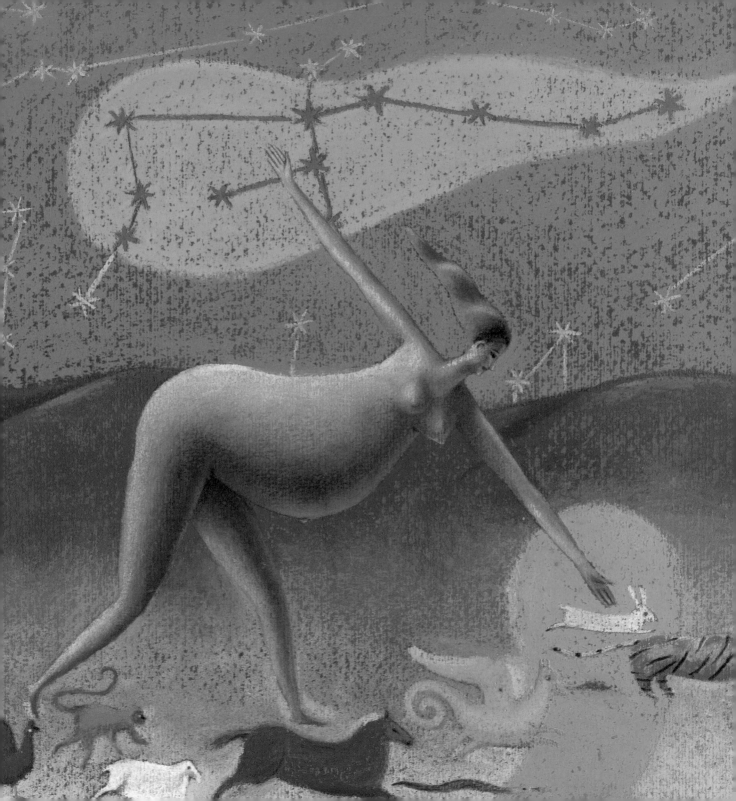

Withchild

WISDOM AND TRADITIONS FOR PREGNANCY,
BIRTH AND MOTHERHOOD

by Deborah Jackson

CHRONICLE BOOKS

SAN FRANCISCO

With Child
Deborah Jackson

First published in the United States in 1999 by Chronicle Books.

Conceived, created and designed by
Duncan Baird Publishers
Sixth floor
Castle House
75–76 Wells Street
London, W1P 3RE

Commissioned artwork: Jamie Bennett, Fabian Negrin, Leigh Wells

Library of Congress Cataloging-in-Publication data available.

ISBN 0-8118-2400-4

Typeset in Nofret and Amazone BT
Printed in Singapore

Distributed in Canada by
Raincoast Books
8680 Cambie Street
Vancouver, B.C. V6P 6M9

1 3 5 7 9 10 8 6 4 2

Chronicle Books
85 Second Street
San Francisco, CA 94105

Web Site: www.chroniclebooks.com

PUBLISHERS' NOTES
The abbreviations CE and BCE have been used in this book.
CE The Common Era (equivalent to AD)
BCE Before the Common Era (equivalent to BC)

Milliliters (ml) have been used throughout for units of fluid measurement.
5ml is equivalent to 1 teaspoon.

The Publishers and author advise that medical advice is sought
before attempting any of the exercises or herbal or other treatments suggested in this book.
They can take no responsibility for any injury, damage or other adverse
effect resulting from following any of the suggestions herein.

In order to avoid any bias, where relevant the use of "he" and "she", when
referring to a baby, alternates topic by topic throughout this book.

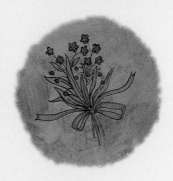

In loving memory of Ben

Contents

Introduction

The future of mothering is a cause for concern in the West. Ancient assumptions about maternal instinct and infant bonding are being eroded by scientists, who tell us that motherhood is little more than a series of chemical reactions and physical cues, enhanced by parenting classes. It seems there's no magic about mothers any more.

After giving birth, preferably with as little sensation as possible, a Western mother is often under pressure to return to "real" work outside the home, where she will be accorded social status and pay. The alternative – staying at home to take care of baby – is often considered to be no more than domestic dawdling, a second-class role that could be undertaken by anyone. Many women feel torn between conflicting roles if they attempt to function both as caring mothers and effective working professionals.

In many parts of the world, despite global advances in science and communication, there are women who are untouched by these debates and conflicts. They do not parent from theory, nor are they aware that motherhood can be a disposable asset. They fulfil a legacy of motherhood that has been handed down for generations, according to ancient matriarchal wisdoms.

In remote regions, tribes manage without the conveniences we take for granted. In places where the most urgent purpose is survival, the task of mothering is regarded in high esteem and mothers themselves are recognized as the essential guardians of life. Parenthood is an elevated role, surrounded with mystery and wonder; it is celebrated with feasts, rituals and offerings and protected with taboos. Raising the next generation is recognized as the most important job of all.

It is difficult to approach the world's diverse mothering practices objectively. Some customs appear delightful, others seem to be no more than superstition, and still others are even seemingly harmful.

This book is not meant to be an uncritical celebration of all things ethnic. Instead, it aims to highlight traditions of the world that celebrate motherhood and gathers together a diverse range of mother's lore, offering insights into the universal subjects of bearing and raising children. Many suggestions on how to adapt these traditions to our own mothering experience are drawn from the world's rich source of practical wisdom. We are given glimpses into cultures which venerate and respect women, allowing us all to remember that there are infinite ways to raise a child, none of which is "correct". And as we celebrate our differences, we may once again feel connected in our common task of raising the children and parents of the future.

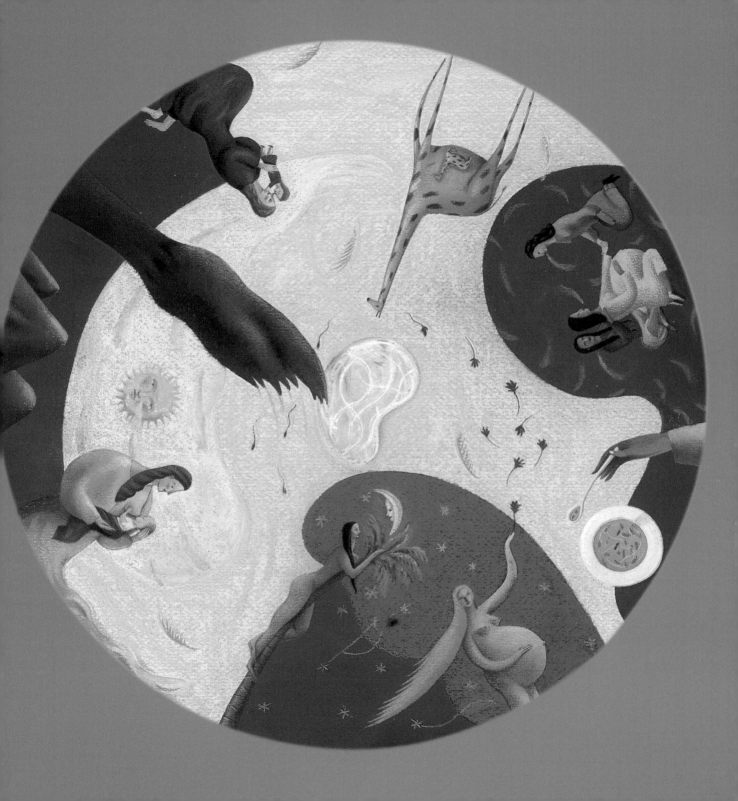

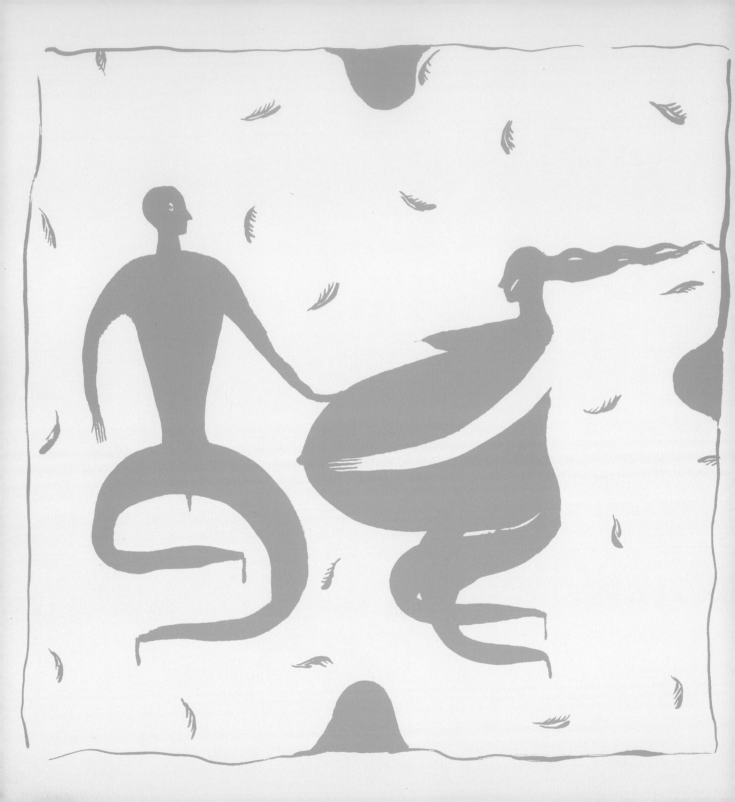

The Time of Promise

Even when we understand the scientific explanation of parenthood, the creation of a new life still fills us with awe and wonder. Fertility and conception retain the deep mystery of the ancient and universal mother goddess, in whose fruitful womb the gift of life is conceived.

The Mother Goddess

Every one of us was carried for nine months – or thereabouts – in the all-embracing comfort of our mother's womb. This simple, universal fact of life probably formed the basis of humanity's earliest religions.

Prehistoric peoples were in awe of the Great Mother, a divine figure from whom all life flowed. Many scholars believe that this female deity of life and fertility may have been the sole object of devotion for our early ancestors. The theory is that, long before complex civilizations emerged with their ranks of household gods, and before the arrival of an all-powerful masculine godhead, there was only one being considered worthy of adoration – the all-giving mother goddess.

Throughout the world, traditions of the divine mother figure tell of her life-giving powers. Aditya, the ancient Iranian goddess who represented vast primordial space, gave birth to seven children, who became the gods of the sun, moon and stars. Bachue, a mother goddess of the Incas, gave birth to the first humans before transforming herself into a snake and returning to the sacred waters of the lake from which she had first emerged.

In Greek mythology, the earth mother Gaia conceived and gave birth by herself to the sky-god Uranus. Their subsequent union produced the first generation of Greek gods (six ferocious Titans and six Titanesses), three Cyclopes and monsters with a hundred hands.

The match between earth mothers and sky fathers is repeated in many ancient religions. In the Maori creation myth, Papa, the earth mother, and Rangi, the sky father, were clasped in an eternal embrace. They held each other so tightly that their unborn children, the gods of nature, were imprisoned in Papa's womb. Tane, the future god of the forests, decided to separate Rangi and Papa. From within the womb, he raised his father sky with his head and pushed his mother earth downward with his

In Chinese myth, the goddess Nu Wa created the first humans from mud, but the task became too great for her: "I can't make mud dolls for ever. Have families and fill the world!"

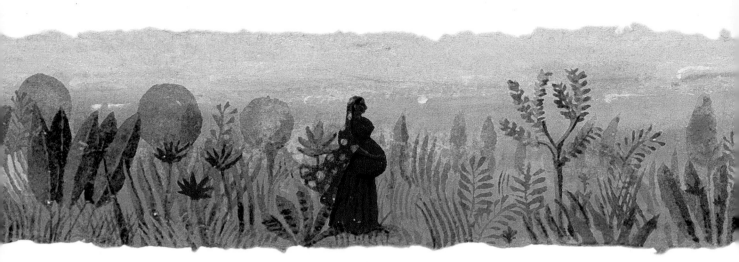

feet. The embrace was released and the gods of nature were born.

Ancient goddesses may have been infinitely fertile – benign archetypes with open arms and ample, child-bearing hips – but the Great Mother also had darker incarnations. She ruled with flashes of brutality as well as generosity of spirit. The Morrigan, a terrifying Celtic goddess in triple form, controlled death and sexuality as well as the forces of life. Her flame-haired figure was sometimes depicted with three heads or even three bodies. In other accounts, the Morrigan was known as Badhbh, meaning "boiling", and was symbolized by a cauldron which bubbled continuously, disgorging all life.

Mother goddesses presided over the thresholds of human experience, ushering babies into existence and shepherding the dying toward the afterlife. They were the objects of both awe and fear, and were often invoked as the final arbiters over the survival of a newly delivered baby or of safely gathered crops. In the Balkans, people still make corn dollies, representing the ancient goddess Nerthus, to ensure a plentiful harvest.

In ancient Rome, Juno (consort and sister of the great god Jupiter) was the guardian of women and childbirth – the equivalent of the Greek deity Hera. While Jupiter was god of the sky and bringer-of-light, Juno was the goddess of the moon and the guardian of all things dark, hidden and female. For the ancient Romans, a woman's *juno*, or protective female spirit, would guide her as she entered a new home, increase her fertility and assist her during pregnancy and labour. It was believed that Juno bestowed the gift of sight on newborn babies.

When the Romans conquered Britain, aspects of the popular Celtic goddess Brigit, protector of women and childbirth, were assimilated into Juno, including the title Queen of Heaven. Brigit was Christianized and regarded as the midwife or foster-mother of Jesus. According to a Hebridean Christian fable, Brigit placed three drops of pure water on the holy infant's brow. This belief was adapted from an older pagan story in which the goddess Brigit bestowed a blessing of triple purity (three drops of wisdom) on the the Son of Light. Scottish Highlanders in the Hebrides used to offer their prayers for safe childbirth to Brigit "the Bride".

Ajysyt, Great Mother to the Siberian Yakut tribe, lived in heaven, writing down the fate of each child in a golden book. She watched over every new baby's birth and brought the baby's soul from heaven, to make the newborn child complete.

Meskhenet, an Egyptian goddess who presided over childbirth, acted as a sacred midwife and was believed to arrange each baby's destiny. Mothers would take their special prayers for a healthy baby to Meskhenet, whose symbol was the birthing tile over which mothers squatted in labour.

Today, mother goddess cults have virtually vanished in the West, but women can rediscover their symbolic power by celebrating their divine foremothers. You could commemorate Yule (December 21), the winter solstice, when mother goddesses such as the Babylonian Ishtar and Astarte traditionally gave birth to the sun. You might observe the Celtic festival of Imbolc – literally "in the womb" – on February 1, to revere the heavily pregnant mother earth. On May Night, you could mark Celtic Beltane (May 1), when the May Queen married the sun god to restore universal harmony, after the upheaval of winter decay and spring regeneration.

Earth and Water

More than 2,500 years ago, the ancient Greeks identified the four elements that they believed were essential to human life: air and fire were male, earth and water female. Earth was the principal element: the provider of shelter and food for all living things.

To our early ancestors, mountains were physical embodiments of mother goddesses and mountain caves were the potent wombs of creation. Childless earth-worshipping women pressed themselves against the ground in the hope of becoming fertile. Ancient Roman women would wash their newborn babies and place them on the ground as a gesture of thanksgiving to the life-giving earth. Even today, caves and rock formations in the shape of the *yoni* (sacred vulva) are worshipped throughout India.

Water, the second female element, was intrinsically linked with fecundity and birth. Early ancestors of the Finns and Hungarians prayed to a Water Mother for babies; while African women traditionally gave birth near rivers and streams, drawing strength from the sound of the rushing water.

Water also symbolizes rebirth: rain regenerates parched soil; baptism marks the beginning of new life; flood myths, common to many cultures, represent the chance to start afresh; fountains and trickling water convey the promise of rejuvenation and growth. Delaware Native Americans venerate Mother Running Water, a river goddess with the power to both bring and take life by fertilizing and flooding the land.

The female elements can provide spiritual sustenance during pregnancy. On a warm day, try walking barefoot in the garden – imagine yourself connecting with mother earth as you do so. Or sit by a river or stream. Close your eyes and listen to the sound that the water makes. Visualize the course of pregnancy as the inexorable current of a flowing river.

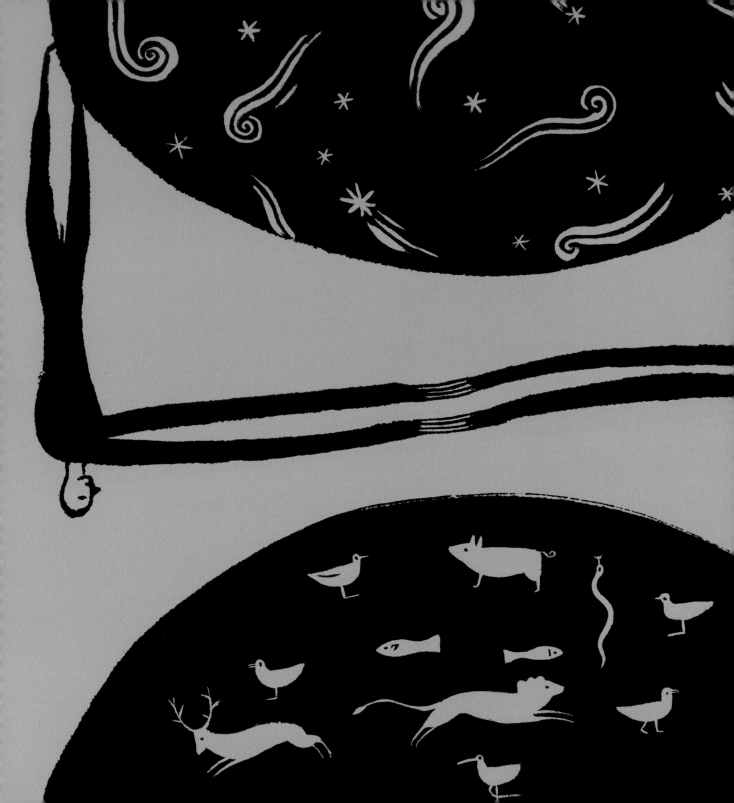

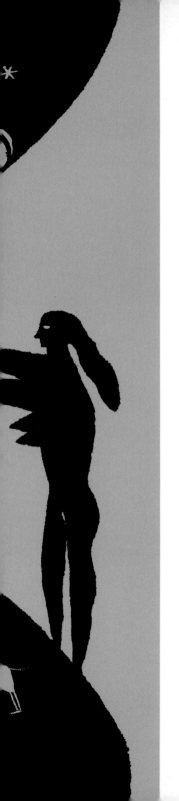

Mother Earth, Father Sky

Weave us clothing of great brightness
That we may walk where birds sing and grass grows green.
Oh, our mother the earth,
Oh, our father the sky.

Prayer of the Teura peoples of New Mexico

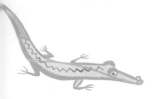

Almost Pregnant

*S*ince ancient times, people have used magic and ritual to summon up the forces of fertility. Celtic Druids gathered acorns at night – when mysterious powers are said to be more potent – to use in their fertility magic. They also carried pine cones as fertility charms. In the Gambia, women washed in sacred crocodile waters to enhance their procreative powers.

Many societies place great significance on child-bearing, and the pressure to conceive can be intense. In the Kayapó tribe of Brazil, adults are ranked according to their fertility and are therefore keen to have children to climb the social ladder. The most respected community members are "fathers (or mothers) of many children". To keep the optimism flowing, a newly married Moroccan bride may reassure relatives that she is "almost pregnant". Moroccan mothers are also protected by the folk tradition of the *ragad*, or "sleeping baby". Married women who continue to menstruate are told that the fetus has fallen asleep in the womb and may

not awaken for up to seven years. This sympathetic fable immediately removes any urgency.

If no children arrive at all, Swahili-speaking people of Chole Island, Tanzania, have their own practical solution: childless couples are given a baby by relatives who have offspring to spare. Up to a quarter of all children are permanently fostered out by the Chole Islanders, who place great importance on having children to look after them in their old age.

Traditional Native American fertility rites, usually involving symbols of fecundity from the natural world, began as soon as a girl reached puberty. Hopi Indian girls dressed their hair in whorls at the side of the head to represent squash blossom – a reproductive symbol. At her wedding, a Hopi woman would wear a headdress shaped like a conch (the shell symbolizing female reproductive organs) and thereafter dressed her hair in braids to resemble ripening ears of corn. Apache girls were presented with a woven basket

An old North American fertility charm assures a married couple that, if they throw cow peas (also called black-eyed peas) across the road near their home, they will become fertile.

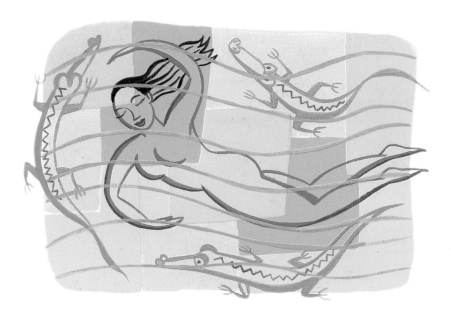

containing sacred pollen at their ritual puberty ceremony.

Modern Western marriages still retain elements of fertility charms, based on the relationship between our fertility and the land. Confetti is a substitute for rice, which was traditionally thrown in the hope that its productivity would encourage conception. Sprays of gypsophila ("baby's breath") in the bridal bouquet also symbolize fecundity. The European custom of tying shoes (thought to represent female reproductive organs) to the back of a wedding car is supposed to herald many children.

A desire for children can be so powerful that in the West fertility is often regarded as a thing to influence rather than as a natural force. When we can control almost every aspect of our lives, it comes as a shock if we do not conceive the moment we intend. It takes an average of six months to conceive – by then around sixty per cent of women will be pregnant. Many more will conceive after a year, and, at two years, ninety per cent will have become pregnant. It may be better to avoid labels like "infertility" and imagine ourselves in the hopeful state of being "almost pregnant".

Conceiving is Believing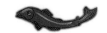

*T*he medical explanation for the wonderful miracle of life often seems inadequate. *Where do babies come from?* is a universal question that has been explained in a huge variety of ways, from euphemisms of baby-producing gooseberry bushes and benevolent storks in the West, to cyclical Buddhist journeys of reincarnated spirits in the East.

In many cultures, conception is more than a biological event – it is a spiritual interaction. For example, Ainu children in Japan are regarded as the physical embodiments of their ancestors' spirits. In Thailand, conception is regarded as the moment when a soul enters a woman's body during intercourse. This soul will have lived many times before and its character will be fully formed. However, the rebirth indicates that it has not yet attained the highest level of disembodied spiritual existence.

For some tribal peoples sex is not considered necessary for conception. Anbarra Aborigines in central Arnhem Land, Australia, say that "spirit children" were placed in certain freshwater pools and water holes during the Dreamtime. Women who want to be pregnant visit areas rumoured to be rich in spirit babies. These beings are rarely seen, for they are said to be as small as walnuts. Each spirit child chooses a mother whom it thinks will be kind, and swims inside her, and in this way she becomes pregnant. Another widespread Aboriginal conception belief is that if a man traps a spirit child in the form of a fish or an animal while hunting and then feeds it to his wife, she will conceive. The resulting child will have certain attributes of the animal's spirit, and even a physical mark corresponding to the place where the animal was speared by the father.

In old England sowing parsley was said to bring babies. When children asked where they came from, they were often told that they came out of the parsley bed.

According to the Dogon people of West Africa, for conception to occur a man must whisper tales of the ancient ancestors into a woman's ear before lovemaking. The words then swirl down to the womb to become the celestial liquid impregnated by the man's essence.

The Greek philosopher Aristotle believed that semen was the sole source of life, but in some societies, such as the Ashanti of West Africa, the father is regarded as superfluous to conception and babies are said to be made from menstrual blood alone.

Women of the Kayapó tribe of Brazil conduct their own impregnation rituals deep in the forest. Standing in a river, stripped to the waist, the woman is brushed with leaves by her friends; they fasten a vine around her waist and she drinks special bark juice. Even though they realize where babies really come from, the women attain a certain amount of sexual freedom through this "forest baby" ritual – women who don't wish to be restricted to one husband say that they are expecting a forest baby, a gift from Mother Nature herself.

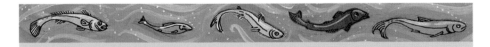

A Sea-voyage Back to Life

The Trobriand Islanders of the South Pacific have one of the most enchanting conception beliefs in the world, which links conception with water. Each newborn child is said to be a rejuvenated spirit who has chosen to journey back to life, across the sea, from the Island of the Dead. The spirit floats back to the islands, clinging to driftwood and sacred seaweed to ease his journey, and a woman conceives by bathing in the ocean and "catching" one of the spirits. The returning spirit itself has no name, but it is believed to rejoin the mother-line of its previous birth.

Fishermen claimed to hear the spirits crying "wa wa" over the waves and, even today, the Trobriand Islanders' word for "fetus" is *waiwaia*, a continual reminder of the spiritual journey of all babies.

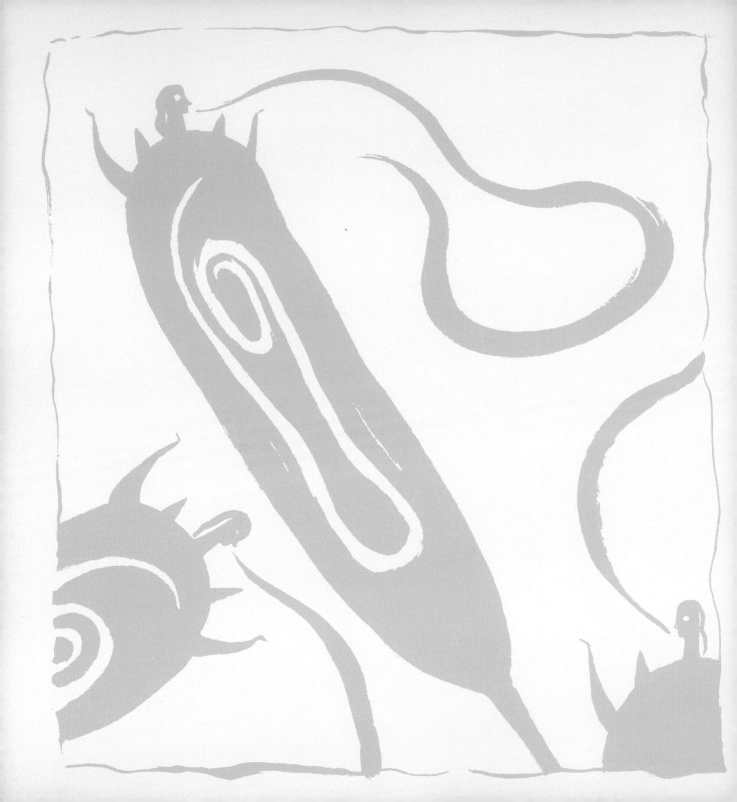

The Child Within

Enclosed in his cocoon, the unborn child is a source

of joy and anticipation. He teases his mother with

fluttering movements and entertains her with dreams

rich in symbols. The nine months of waiting are a chance

to prepare body and mind for the completely new focus

of motherhood. As you eat, breathe and move,

you do so on another's behalf.

Mysteries of Gender

*I*f a Jamaican woman sees shoals of fish swimming through her dreams, she takes it as a sign that a baby is probably on the way – but still the question remains, will the baby be a boy or girl? All over the world, people look for signs of the baby's sex. If we are to believe gender myths from numerous cultures, the baby's sex can be determined at any time throughout pregnancy – and even before it.

The Greek philosopher Aristotle promoted the belief that a man's right testicle produced boys while his left created girls. Thus, men in ancient Greece who wanted sons often had their left testicle tied up and, in some extreme cases, removed altogether.

In ancient Mexico, it was believed that the "nature essence" of either the mother or father would determine the child's sex during intercourse. As the parents made love, the mouth of the uterus was said to open and a drop of blood would fall into it

from either parent. If the first drop was the mother's blood, the baby would be a boy; if the father's, a girl would be born.

Many gender divination techniques concentrate on the mother's appearance and actions, or the things that happened to her, during pregnancy. In some cultures it is believed that the baby's sex can not only be determined at this time, but influenced too – if the mother-to-be behaves in a certain way she can encourage nature to bring her a boy or a girl as is her wish.

In Bihar, northeastern India, if an expectant mother crosses any threshold, into and out of a room or building, with her left foot first, the action is believed to bring a baby girl; with the right foot, it is said to bring a boy. As in many other cultures (today, as well as in the past), the Biharis favour the birth of sons over daughters. As a result, an expectant Bihar mother spends her pregnancy entering and leaving rooms with her right foot first.

In Hungary, eastern Europe, it is believed that, if a pregnant woman wishes to bear a son, she should place seeds from a poppy on the window sill of her home. If she would prefer to have a girl, she must sprinkle sugar grains there instead.

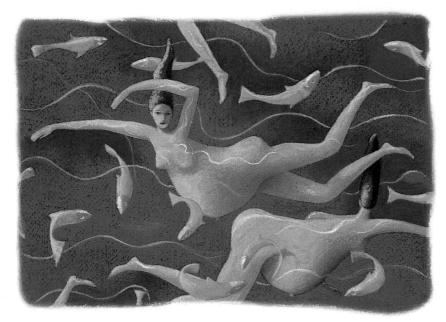

Gender speculation has grown up mostly because many cultures had an inevitable curiosity about the unborn child. The widespread belief that the continuation of the male line was paramount, may have encouraged people to try to discover whether their newborn would be that all–important boy. In southern Africa, Zulu mothers say that if a green or black snake appears in the home-stead, the newborn will be a boy, while the appearance of a puff-adder signifies a girl.

The mother's appearance is also supposed to give clues to the gender of the baby. The ancient Greek physi-cian Hippocrates believed that the left eye and left breast were bigger in a woman who was expecting a baby girl – the opposite, of course, for a baby boy. Native North Americans looked for tiny fish–hook symbols in the whites of a woman's eyes – roughly at the four– and eight-o'clock positions beneath her irises. Fish–hook shapes in the right eye were said to signify a girl; in the left, a boy. (If hooks could be seen in both eyes it was said that the woman was expecting twins, or simply that she already had children.)

Indigenous peoples of ancient Mexico, and the Nyinba people of Nepal, once believed that boys lay on the right-hand side of the uterus and girls on the left.

In England women today follow an old-wives' tale that boys are carried in front, and girls are carried more broadly, around the sides and front, wrapping themselves closer to their mothers for protection (while boys strive for independence).

Among the Dusin of northern Borneo, parents-to-be believe that a boy fetus moves quickly and roughly, while a girl moves quietly and gently. The Hamar people of southern Ethiopia understand that whenever *Barjo*, or Fate, creates a new human being, if the child smiles at the moment of birth, she becomes a woman, and if not he becomes a man.

If you are curious to test the accuracy of a particular ancient prediction device, try an ever-popular test that originated among the Romany people of Hungary. This method of gender speculation was (and still is) practised throughout the whole of Europe. 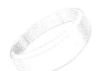 Prop yourself up on cushions, either on a sofa, a bed, or on the floor, so that you feel comfortable. Lie back with your legs stretched out in front of you and your stomach (and the baby) facing skyward. Take a deep breath and relax. Ask a member of your family or a close friend to tie a pure gold ring (most appropriately your wedding ring if you have one) onto a length of string or cotton, and hold it suspended high above your stomach. Your prediction partner should lower the ring slowly toward your unborn baby and, as he or she does so, the ring should start to move. A strong, circular movement is said to indicate that you are carrying a baby girl; a swing from side to side, like the movement of a pendulum, is said to indicate that the baby is a boy.

Of course, it really makes no difference what the signs and portents are, as the gender of a baby is determined from the moment that the sperm meets the egg and is beyond our control. Our role is not to change our developing baby, but to welcome and cherish whoever he or she may turn out to be.

Dream Babies

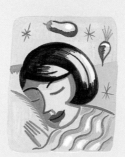

In cultures where a child's sex may be of great importance to the expectant parents, the symbols in a pregnant woman's dreams are closely examined for gender clues. Across many diverse cultures, dream gender symbols tend to fall into two distinct groups: round objects are believed to symbolize a female child and long, phallic-shaped objects are thought to suggest that a male child is on the way.

For example, Nyinba women of Nepal suspect that they are carrying a boy if they dream of long vegetables, such as radishes or aubergines. (They also say that cutting tools, traditionally male implements, indicate a boy.) Alternatively, they say that "girl" dreams feature round vegetables (as well as prayer beads and other circular objects). If a New Zealand Maori mother-to-be dreamed of a human skull, she would have traditionally taken this as an indication that she was carrying a girl; dreams of feathers, on the other hand, would have suggested a boy.

In modern societies in the West, a child's sex may not be a matter of great importance to the parents. However, pregnancy dreams can still be interpreted as indicators of a mother's hopes and expectations for her future child. For example, it is common to dream of a baby who is imperfect in some way. Facing up to this possibility in your dreams is your mind's way of preparing you for some of the uncontrollable aspects of motherhood.

Try writing a dream diary during pregnancy. As soon as you wake up, jot down your dreams in a notepad. Try to interpret your dream images in the context of your waking life. Over time, your own personal patterns of dream symbolism, and your unspoken feelings about your child, will emerge.

Movement and Meditation

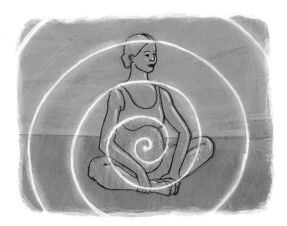

Yoga's Tailor Pose helps to soften ligaments during pregnancy (ask your doctor to advise you at what stages it is safe for you to exercise). After a warm bath, sit on the floor with your back straight and bring the soles of your feet together in front of you. Breathing deeply, slowly draw your feet toward your body. With each out-breath, relax the hips and spine. Allow your knees to open out toward the floor.

Tongan women believe that staying in any position for too long will make birth harder – you can prepare your body for the physical task of labour by taking regular exercise during pregnancy, although *always* consult your doctor before you begin any physical activity. Bedouin women live by the motto "toil hard, walk far", working outside and riding camels right up until the hour of birth. Pregnant women in New Guinea have specially designed obstacle courses, while in Sanpoil, India, mothers-to-be run and swim their way to fitness. Swimming is usually ideal during pregnancy as your body (and your unborn baby) is supported by the water. Although it might seem strange, belly dancing can help to prepare the pelvis and abdominal muscles for birth. Once known as *la danse du ventre* ("womb dancing"), its undulations and squatting movements represent conception and birth.

With Babies in Mind

"Think beautiful thoughts" is an age-old prescription for pregnancy, but not always easy to do in a stressful world. Take time out, as pregnant women in China and Japan used to do, for a daily meditation with your baby – a simple and beneficial way to begin the subtle bonding process.

Sit comfortably and slow your breathing. You could try a Zulu pregnancy breathing exercise before beginning to meditate: take three consecutive in-breaths so that your lungs are completely filled with air, and then one long out-breath to expel negative thoughts (in your mind's eye watch them disappearing) and energize your body. You may find that your baby starts to move as you tune in, or if you play familiar music softly in the background. Visualize her small body and sense her, warm and protected, in the amniotic fluid. Spend a few minutes in open awareness. When you become skilled at harnessing your mind's energies, you can use them later to ease birth.

Visualize a place where you can be happy and alone – a garden, for example. Look around at the flowers and enjoy the tranquillity. When you are ready, walk further into your picture, down some steps, perhaps, into a secluded courtyard. Water trickles from fountains, and birds swoop and sing. Affirm the positive messages you will need to hear during labour: your body opens easily and painlessly, each contraction bringing your baby closer. Finally, turn and walk up the steps, through your garden and back into the moment.

Practise finding your inner refuge in this way throughout pregnancy, perhaps using a physical trigger, such as clasping your hands.

A Sensory Connection

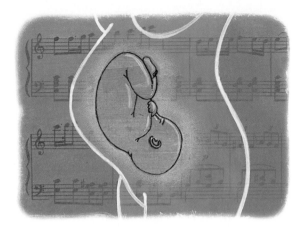

Some people say that a new baby cannot feel pain. But still, even in the womb his senses are highly

alert. For example, his ears are adjusted so that through the amniotic fluid he is able to hear his

mother's heartbeat and some of the sounds from outside her body, modulated by a liquid world.

Sensory perception is highly developed in the womb. A baby's skin, so smooth and sensitive, is protected by fine hair and a layer of grease (vernix). Babies also have a wonderful capacity for taste, with tastebuds all over the mouth and tongue, tens of thousands more than they will have at ten years old.

The sense that most connects the unborn baby with the outside world is his ability to hear. As the mother talks to her child, she imprints herself on his brain, making a pre–natal bond that will continue throughout his life. In the Congo, pregnant women sing to their unborn children. The same song is repeated over and over throughout pregnancy to allow the baby to associate the sound with security and comfort. Then, once the baby is born, the mother sings the song to her baby again. The familiar sound is immediately comforting to the child, who is calmed by the way in which it resonates through the bombardment of mysterious and bewildering sounds in his new world outside the womb.

Happiness Outside and In

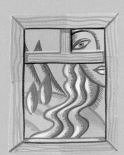

Some people believe that, just as sounds can filter from the outside world into the womb and be heard by the unborn baby, emotions and thoughts can be transferred, too. It is almost as if external actions and reactions can be seen by the baby through his own secret window on the world.

In Thailand an unborn child is thought to react to all the stimuli that affect his mother. As a result, she takes great care to have only positive experiences throughout her pregnancy. A pregnant Thai woman is also careful never to watch another woman giving birth. It is believed that, through his mother's eyes, the baby being born would be embarrassed to be "watched" by another baby, and that the baby "watching" would be embarrassed by what he sees. It is said that, as a consequence, both babies would refuse to be born easily.

Elsewhere some mothers put pressure on their families and their friends to improve their behaviour so that the unborn child learns only good and decent human actions, which he will then take into his own life.

The idea that the mother's happiness in turn influences the mood of the unborn baby is related in an ancient story that blends both Christian and pagan traditions. Before the infant Christ was born, Mary and Joseph visited a wonderful cherry orchard. Taken by the beauty of one of the trees and the delicious looking fruit, Mary asked her husband to pick her a cherry, but Joseph refused. Mary became sad and this melancholy was sensed by the unborn Christ who, desperate for his mother's happiness, bade the tree bow down its branches to offer fruit to Mary. As it did so, Mary's happiness, and that of her baby, were restored.

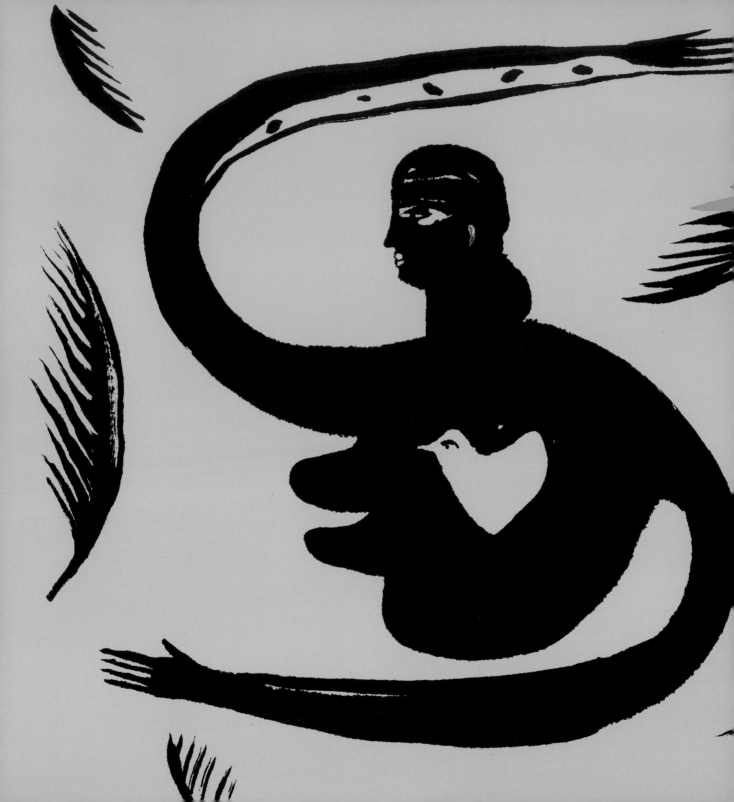

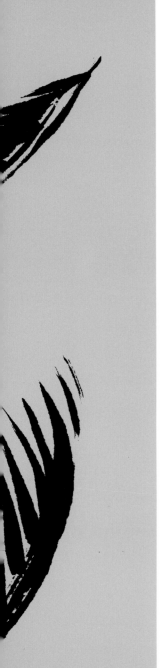

My Heart Flies

My heart is so joyous,
My heart flies in singing.
Under the trees of the forest,
The forest, our home, our mother.
In my net I have caught
A little bird,
A very little bird,
And my heart is caught
In the net with the little bird.

Pregnancy song of the Efé peoples

Calming the Waves

Pregnancy is supposed to be a time of "blooming" when women become visions of radiant beauty. Many mothers-to-be do exude health and happiness, especially in the middle months, but there may well be times when you feel more like wilting.

Waves of tiredness and nausea are often the first signs of pregnancy; in countries where tests are unavailable, women welcome these symptoms as proof that they are truly pregnant.

Nevertheless, every culture has its own preferred remedy for "morning sickness". In Indonesia, women drink the juice of a young coconut. If the sickness is very bad, a midwife uses prayers and incantations to give the juice supernatural healing powers. In Austria, mothers drink cups of fennel tea, while in Japan they eat the flesh of an Umeboshi plum.

In ancient Rome, pregnant women started the day with a drink of water infused with cinnamon and lime juice. Other nausea-calming teas are ginger (grate one teaspoon of fresh ginger root into a cup of hot water and let it steep for five minutes) or dried orange peel (grate and dry the peel of an organic orange, then steep the peel in hot water for twenty minutes). A few drops of chamomile flower essence in water is an all-round pregnancy pick-me-up, easing nausea and stomach upsets, calming emotions and inducing restful sleep. Early nights and lots of healthy snacks also help.

The ancient Egyptians pioneered the use of herbal medicine and essential oils, used in the West today to alleviate common pregnancy discomforts. However, you must seek advice from your doctor as certain oils, such as sage and myrrh, should never be used while you are pregnant. During pregnancy your skin needs extra care – after all, it has to stretch to accommodate your growing baby. But skin is a remarkably elastic material and, although stretch marks can appear fairly indiscriminately, by taking care of your skin during pregnancy you can help to reduce the tell-tale signs. Massage your skin with a mixture of

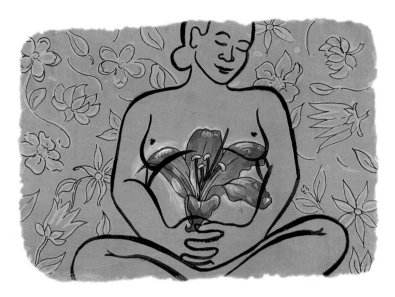

3 drops each of wheatgerm, borage seed and carrot oils in 50ml of almond oil. A wonderful evening massage mixture is 20 drops of lavender oil (a good sleep-aid) and 3 drops of neroli in 50ml of almond oil. Using light, sweeping movements, gently rub the oils into your skin. Massage your skin regularly during pregnancy and also for a few months after birth. In traditional societies, pregnant women meet their midwives for a tender massage and have soothing preparations rubbed into their skin, from warm kukai oil in Hawaii to coconut oil in Malaysia. Cocoa butter and almond oil are also widely used.

To help prevent varicose veins, massage your legs with a mixture of 2 drops of geranium oil and 2 drops of lemon oil in 50ml of almond oil. Acupuncture, the ancient Chinese healing art which stimulates the release of energy blockages, can also be used to ease swollen veins, as well as backache. Traditional remedies for heartburn (common in late pregnancy) include: peppermint tea; a drop of rose oil on sugar; chewing almonds with orange peel; eating fresh papaya after meals; or the ancient Indian cure of a drop of sandalwood oil with sugar, or dissolved in honey water (taken before you go to bed).

Food for Life

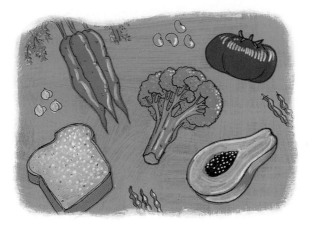

A baby's organs are formed entirely during the first trimester, so it is clearly important for expectant mothers to eat well from conception. Food scientists have trouble defining optimum pregnancy nutrition. They used say eat liver, now they say avoid it. Currently in vogue are oily fish (research from Denmark suggests that babies are born heavier), folic acid (from green, leafy vegetables) and even certain curries.

Stand under a mango tree and eat a mango. If you are expecting a baby, the fruit will taste like anything but mango. This traditional pregnancy test from the Philippines reveals a fascinating feature of the antenatal state.

Hormone production often makes the saliva taste metallic, which alters our sense of taste – even old favourites like coffee or tea may become unpalatable. As you start to reject your favourite foods, you might also experience strange cravings. In Nepal, the Nyinba tribe believe that if a woman craves spicy food, she will have a girl; if she craves bland food, a boy is expected. Some women eat one unusual food to excess; others are drawn to comforting nursery foods like porridge or rice pudding. A classic non-food craving is for coal, which can indicate mineral deficiency. Do not be alarmed if you suddenly realize that you want a banana and onion pizza – your body is literally catering to its needs.

Eating for Two

Babies develop in the womb on a huge variety of foods, from a traditional Inuit mother's regimen of whale blubber and fish to a Yoruba vegetarian diet. There is no single ideal diet but wholesome fresh food and a balance of nutrients are important.

"Eating for two" does not mean eating twice the amount of food, but you do need increased levels of certain nutrients, especially calcium and iron. In the last three months of pregnancy, some doctors recommend increased calcium intake. Dairy products are excellent sources of calcium and green vegetables, such as spinach, are rich in iron. Ask your doctor for advice.

Food restrictions are plentiful in every culture and involve more than just the nutritional characteristics of food. Filipino women avoid eating "twin" bananas (believed to cause twins); Thai mothers eat "cooling" bananas to ensure that their babies are not hot-tempered; African mothers say that eggs, milk and meat cause "hot blood" – increased sexual desire – and as sex is believed to harm the baby in the later months of pregnancy, these sources of protein are avoided.

Food observance is often part of an elaborate preparation for a smooth delivery. Tagalog women in the Philippines eat lots of eggs during pregnancy to make the baby slip out easily. The Yukaghir Siberian nomads avoid eating the fat of a cow, reindeer or larch gum tree as these substances are said to thicken inside the woman and fasten her baby to the walls of the womb. Lepcha women in the Himalaya do not eat rice that has stuck to the pan, as it is said to make the placenta stick.

Seven-month Ceremonies

At seven months an unborn child is almost fully formed in the womb, with eyelashes and her own unique fingerprints. She can swallow, suck her thumb, hiccup, hear sounds in the world beyond the womb, and even recognize her mother's voice. All over the world, among indigenous peoples, the seventh month of pregnancy is marked by special ceremonies to rejoice in the new life unfurling.

Holding your own seven-month ceremony is a good way to celebrate your imminent motherhood and the growing vigour of your child. You might devise your own private "walk-about", introducing the child to favourite places, or to the elements (represented by wind, sun, earth and water). In a ritual followed by the Quiché people of Guatemala, a mother describes the scene out loud to her unborn child (you could voice the words in your head if you prefer) and tells her about the woods, rivers and mountains. You could even make your journey within the confines of your own home, taking the baby on a walk through the house, describing each room, what happens there and who spends time in it. You could introduce your baby to members of your family through photographs and share with her the relationships and memories that these represent.

Alternatively, you might consider making a symbolic commitment to the future. If it is autumn, for example, you might choose a special place in your garden and plant seven bulbs that will flower in the spring of your baby's arrival.

Feasting plays a part in many seven-month rituals – most notably in Indonesia. The traditional Javanese feast takes place in the home of the maternal grandmother-to-be, emphasizing the wisdom and experience of childbirth passing down through generations of women. The table is laid with seven pyramids of rice to represent the seven months of pregnancy; eight or nine balls of rice to symbolize the saints who brought Islam to Indonesia; and a large rice pyramid, believed to give symbolic strength to the baby. In Indonesia the child in the womb is thought of as a mystic meditating in a cave, strengthening herself spiritually for her emergence into the world.

In many ceremonies, the guests perform symbolic tasks associated with the birth to come. Father, midwife, mother-in-law, friends – all have parts to play, beginning the network of support that will guide the child through life. You could easily devise a ceremony of this kind to help mark the turning-point before the more tiring, final months of pregnancy and the countdown to birth. In the box below are a few ideas that you may like to try or adapt for your own seven-month feast.

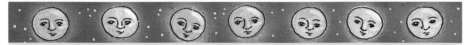

Time for a Feast

An appealing feature of seven-month festivals is a meal to welcome friends and relatives into the company of the unborn child. Holding your own seven-month feast allows those you love to share in your celebration. You could heighten the symbolism in various ways – for example, by hosting a dinner or lunch for seven people, perhaps asking each guest to bring along a dish. In the centre of the table you might set seven candles, perhaps held in a *menorah* – a sacred candelabrum, from Jewish tradition, with seven stems representing, among other things, the seven branches of the Tree of Life.

As a souvenir of the occasion, your guests could sign a special record book where everyone, including yourself, writes a personal message to your child.

The Unfolding Lotus

Ripe fruit is plucked easily from a tree. But how do we know when a baby is ready to come? Contractions may begin in slow waves, as if the child is waking from a deep sleep. Waters breaking is a sure sign that labour is beginning. But rarely does labour start with panic and frenzied puffing, as we might imagine.

In Malaysia, midwives feel a woman's feet as she nears her time. When the big toe grows cold, it means that body heat is shifting toward the womb, ready for labour. Once her ankles lose heat, birth is imminent. (Japanese women are advised to wear socks to "keep baby cosy".)

Every culture has its own ways of preparing for labour and easing the baby's arrival. A Thai woman eats lotus buds blessed by a Buddhist monk, so that her body will open like the lotus flower. According to classic Chakra (energy-centre) meditation, the crown of the head is a thousand-petalled lotus unfolding toward the divine energy of the universe. During birth, Indian women borrow this image to visualize the cervix opening with each contraction – and you can do the same.

Traditional birth lore concentrated on apt symbolism, which often involved undoing knots at every opportunity. African women do not plait their hair during pregnancy, and Navaho Native Americans avoid hanging out washing, as they say that this action causes knots in the umbilical cord.

Many birth treatments are suggestively slippery, symbolically willing the baby to slither out easily. Before labour Cherokee mothers take a ritual bath infused with slippery bark; they also take a powerful herb to make the baby "jump down briskly". In the Yemen, the midwife feeds a mother oil and milk to ease the baby's journey. In ancient Mexico, women wore lucky charms – amulets that were made of snail shells to ensure that the baby slipped out as easily as a snail peeks out from its shell.

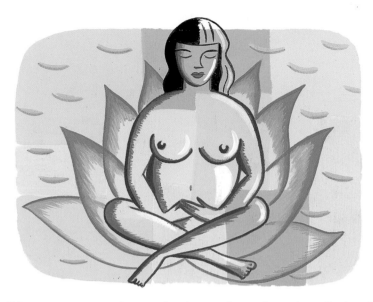

Other treatments, such as perineal massage, are more practical. In the weeks leading up to birth, after a bath, massage the area around the vagina with almond oil – adding 5 drops of rose oil if you like. During labour, a skilled midwife can give an internal massage before the baby has fully descended the birth canal. Some midwives perfect this to the point where tearing is extremely rare, and cutting can be completely unnecessary.

Raspberry leaf tea was traditionally taken by Native North Americans to tone the uterus and dilate pelvic muscles. It is high in vitamin C, which helps to relax tissues, reducing stretch marks and tearing. During labour itself, the tea brings pain relief and helps to expel the placenta. Because of this latter property, you should consult a doctor or herbalist about when it is safe to drink raspberry leaf tea. It can also be used (lukewarm) to wash the baby's eyes after birth – but again always check with your doctor first.

Anthropologists, keen to observe childbirth in tribal societies, may live for months with Inuit or African peoples and never arrive in time for a delivery. "Primitive" birth conditions may not have the benefits of technical wizardry, but normal births are often fast and seemingly effortless.

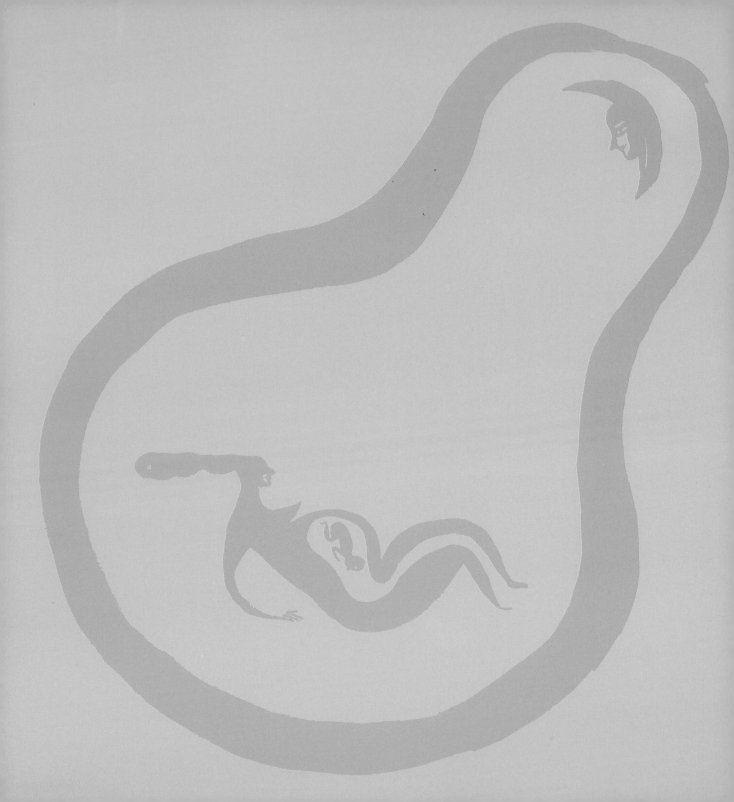

Into the World

World culture has developed myriad traditions to express
the sacred significance of birth. Special consideration for
the place of birth, blessings bestowed by a midwife upon the
newborn, rituals such as burying the placenta, and celestial
birth charts, all represent the culmination of nine months
of passionate anticipation and express our profound
hope for each precious new life.

Birthplace, Birthspace

*W*here is it best to give birth? For many women in the West, hospital is perceived as the safest place (particularly for a first birth), on account of its monitoring equipment and staff specially trained to spot and handle problems. But many women around the world give birth safely outside a hospital environment. Given a choice, the simple answer may be wherever you feel safe and happy.

Despite the proliferation of hospital birth centres, eight out of ten babies in the world are born at home. This may be in a specially allotted room, a space with spiritual and emotional significance. Or it may be the bedroom, often where the baby was actually conceived, and a place of obvious privacy.

In many parts of the world, women return to the home of their own mother in order to give birth, where they can be separate, safe and protected by those who know and love them best. Among the Basuto of Lesotho, a couple's first child actually "belongs" to the maternal grandparents and so is delivered in their house. In many African societies the ancestral spirits said to dwell in the grandmother's hut are believed to protect the mother and child during birth.

A widespread preparation for labour is the stopping up of holes and windows in the birthing room, which is said to keep out evil spirits. The effect is also to create a womb-like area, protected from prying eyes.

Most mothers seek seclusion, often in the familiarity of their own home, for this intimate act, but in some cultures birth was kept away from the home because the blood of childbirth was believed to pollute the household. Japanese women traditionally delivered their babies in small birthing sheds; in Smolensk births took place in a barn; and Arapesh women of New Guinea still give birth in special huts outside the village, to avoid "polluting" the community with childbirth.

There are cultures in which childbirth is a major social event.

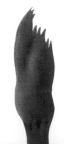

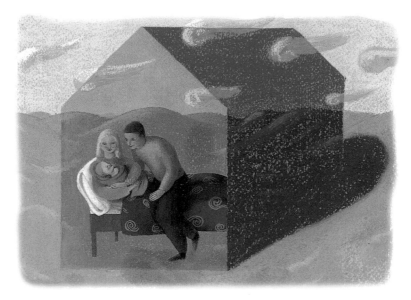

When Navaho Native American mothers go into labour, the whole tribe gathers round to eat a meal and enjoy the spectacle. Among the Basque people of Spain, a mother in labour is traditionally attended by her whole family. Weather permitting, the birth takes place outside, near a running stream. There is a festival atmosphere, with singing, dancing, storytelling and jokes to "massage the mother and baby with laughter".

Yemenite women expect their neighbours and friends to visit during labour, to lend moral support, chant prayers to Allah and help out if necessary. In Yucatán, Maya women in labour are not isolated from day-to-day life. They give birth in hammocks in their one-roomed houses. A blanket is slung from the rafters for a little privacy, but this does not deter their friends from calling by to chat, or animals from wandering in and out. The calm atmosphere of normality helps to alleviate tension.

In places where childbirth was acknowledged as the most important and sacred human act, people designed their houses and villages with birth in mind. Extended Inuit families lived in a karmak, or semi-underground earth house, entered by a low, sloping passageway. As the

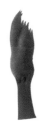

karmak was symbolically associated with the womb, great care was taken to smooth the walls of the entrance, probably to ensure smooth births. Smaller Inuit igloos were designed according to similar principles. Fitting of the final keystone was vital – it had to be as large as possible, in order to make delivery easier. Inside Inuit igloos, areas for men and women were set apart: the floor was given to the men and their hunting tools; while elevated platforms, covered with animal skins and mats, were allotted to women as the place to give birth.

The Dogon people of Mali still build the women's domain and birthing room at the heart of their villages. The door represents the female reproductive organs and the ceiling symbolizes a protectively arched male body. At the time of conception, the new baby's spirit begins its nine-month wait in the women's domain. When the newborn arrives he can collect his spirit immediately upon entering the world.

In medieval Europe, noble women retreated to a special lying-in chamber for the weeks preceding and after birth. A noble woman would choose her own bed covers, wall-hangings and drapes and the room would be equipped with an altar where Mass could be said. Only her husband, priest and ladies-in-waiting were permitted entrance to the lying-in chamber.

Zulu women decorated the birth place with beads and carvings so that the newborn's eyes would fall immediately upon objects of beauty. Thai women festoon their houses with religious tokens – protective cloths painted with magical letters and pictures – to keep away the malevolent spirits that are said to gather around the birth room.

If you have planned where you will give birth, why not transform it into a personalized birthing domain? Scented candles will create a calm atmosphere; inspirational pictures, such as those of happy family occasions, will help positive visualizations; an upstairs room, with a view of the sky, rooftops or hills will give you a sense of space and freedom.

"She reclined, propped up with fair cushions of crimson damask with gold, and was wrapped about with a round mantle of crimson velvet furred with ermine."

An onlooker's view of Jane Seymour, queen to Henry VIII of England, in the room where she gave birth to Edward VI.

Waters of Life

In New Guinea a Gahuku mother gives birth on a river-bank, attended by women who bathe her back and shoulders. The sight and sound of water help concentration, and the flowing stream is said to encourage the movement of the child within.

Water is a universal birth aid, used directly for its soothing and cleansing properties and also as a birth stimulant. To soften the perineum, African mothers labour over steaming hot rocks, and Guatemalan midwives give relaxing steam-bath massages. In the Middle Ages, Finnish women laboured in smoke saunas, where bathhouse midwives called upon water spirits for help.

You could create your own steam room for the early stages of labour. Close the door of your bathroom and fill the bath with hot water. Don't get into the bath. Instead, sit comfortably propped up on cushions on the floor and enjoy the enveloping moist air.

Actually giving birth in water, which has become popular in the West, was rare until this century. Japanese women in remote fishing villages once gave birth in the sea and it is thought that Maoris occasionally had aquatic births.

During a modern waterbirth, immersion is used in the first stages of labour to relieve pain and to stimulate cervical dilation. In fact, one of the greatest gifts of warm water comes from stepping out of it. As you encounter the cool air, labour speeds up, sometimes setting off the "fetus ejection reflex". A newborn baby can survive underwater for up to forty minutes, so you can stay in the birthing tub to give birth. (Consult your doctor about this.) As soon as the baby is born, he should be gently brought to the surface to take his first breath of air.

Catching Babies

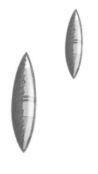

*B*irth is a bridge from one world to the next, and the mother and child making this journey can be vulnerable travellers. Benin African women prefer to give birth alone – to prove their resilience and power – but this is a rare example. On every continent, women turn to midwives to help them reach the other side.

A midwife's role does not always end with "catching babies", as Amish people call it. Traditional midwifery offers a continuous line of care, beginning before pregnancy and culminating with lifelong friendship. In Guatemala a *comadrona*, often a family friend, gives massage for period pains, works as a midwife and has long-term responsibility for the baby. She is part health-professional, part godmother – someone whose concern extends to the spiritual as well as the medical.

Before it came to be treated as a medical condition, childbirth used to be a solely female concern. In English the word "midwife" is derived from the Anglo-Saxon phrase meaning simply "with woman". This principle

of female solidarity is illustrated by the Efé peoples in the rainforest of the Congo. At the onset of labour, two midwives accompany the mother to the river. They sing with her during contractions and, as she squats at the water's edge, they support her on each side, breathing deeply. As the baby's head crowns, the midwives hold their breath and the baby is born. Jean-Pierre Hallet, who, during the 1900s, lived with the Efé on and off for sixty years, described the occasion as a "tremendous feeling of oneness".

Midwives were traditionally honoured as guardians of vital knowledge and skill – the French word for midwife is *sage-femme* ("wise woman"). In many cultures, she is known simply as "grandmother" – not necessarily the mother's mother, but a woman who has experienced generations of childbirth and is revered by the whole community. The African-American "granny midwife" helped to deliver babies and dispensed bitter herbs and root teas for everyday ailments. In many African societies a

"You are a midwife: you are assisting at someone else's birth. Do good without show or fuss ... If you must take the lead, lead so that the mother is helped, yet still free and in charge. When the baby is born, the mother will rightly say: "We did it ourselves!"

Dao De Jing, 500BCE

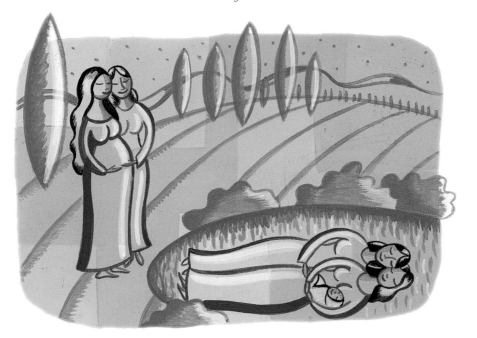

woman becomes a grandmother with any act of midwifery.

Tribal midwives are often regarded as mediators between the spirit and human worlds. They offer incantations and prayers to ensure a safely delivered baby. For the Dinka people of the Sudan, the midwife is known as *geem*, receiver of God's gift of a child. She is the spiritual mother of the newborn, a relationship that the child will honour throughout her life.

Traditional midwifery can be heavy work. In Mexico, a Tzotzil Indian woman gives birth standing up, while a midwife supports her around the waist from behind. During a traditional hammock birth, a Maya midwife is accompanied by helpers who rub the woman's abdomen, back and legs; a "head helper", with her arms under the woman's shoulders, provides extra support during contractions.

After a baby is born, we should not forget to thank the midwives who gave us the courage and strength to give birth. In rural Bulgaria, "Baba", the granny midwife, has her own festival, *Babin Den*, "Grandmother's

Day". Baba was said to impart wisdom to each baby she delivered, and grateful families reward- ed her with flowers. In some Western countries, mothers still thank the mid- wife with a box of chocolates – the heavier the baby, the bigger the box is likely to be.

In places where childbirth has become a more clinical procedure, where women are surrounded by men in white coats, the traditional midwife's role has dimin- ished. Long gone are the days, as in Germany in 1552, when a male doctor might be condemned to death for disguising him- self as a woman to witness childbirth. Perhaps, though, there is a lesson to be learned about the benefits of having women helping women: a traditional Maya midwife says that babies come "like a jet", while many male obstetricians find themselves dealing with long labours.

A Gaelic Midwife's Blessing

The little drop of the Sky, on thy little forehead, beloved one.
The little drop of the Land, on thy little forehead, beloved one.
The little drop of the Sea, on thy little forehead, beloved one.
To aid thee from the fays, to guard thee from the host;
To aid thee from the gnome, to shield thee from the spectre;
To keep thee for the Three, to shield thee, to surround thee;
To save thee for the Three, to fill thee with the graces;
The little drop of the Three, to lave thee with the graces.

Women Who Help Women

Peek inside any maternity ward, and you'll see that technical wizardry has overtaken the intuitive role of the experienced midwife. But there are still ways for mothers to find the human touch. In the USA, *doula* birth companions (*doula* is an ancient Greek term meaning a woman who helps women) are being introduced into hospitals to assist mothers during labour and afterwards. Similar schemes operate in Europe. In ancient Greece *doulas* were handmaidens, often slaves, who were lifelong attendants to their mistresses, and knew them better than anyone else. It followed naturally that, for an ancient Greek woman, her *doula* was the most valued and trusted birth companion.

These days *doulas* are far from being slaves – they are carefully trained professionals who can help a mother to realize that her birth experience is the most natural thing in the world, despite the unfamiliar changes in and reactions of her body. We cannot always choose our midwife, but, whether we intend to be in hospital or at home, we can choose our birth companion. *Doulas* are trained to help you make the best choices about the kind of birth you want to have; to support you throughout labour (and also during pregnancy if you wish); to guide a new father; and to help you care for your new baby for the first few months. Research has shown that a *doula*-assisted birth is as much as fifty percent less likely to result in Caesarean section. Moreover, forceps deliveries and necessary pain relief are also reduced, and mothers are more likely to treat their new babies with sensitivity and warmth. In other words, the *doula's* familiar face and female wisdom might be just the tonic that birthing women need to help them to have an enjoyable and trouble-free birth.

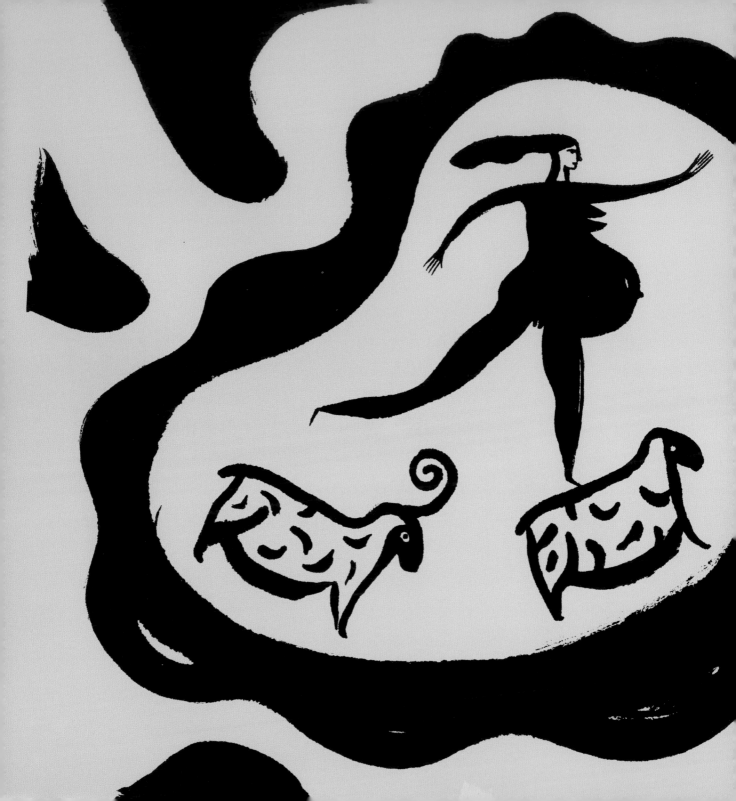

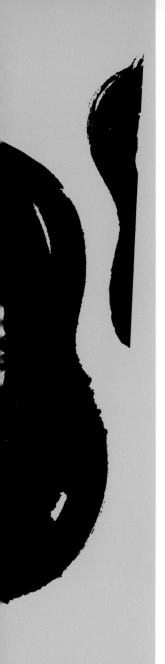

Goats Have No Midwives

Goats have no midwives,
Sheep have no midwives.
When the goat is pregnant, she is safely delivered,
When the sheep is pregnant, she is safely delivered,
You, in this state of pregnancy, will be safely delivered.

Song of the African Yoruba midwife

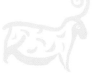

Easing the Way

Navaho Indians have two words to describe labour: one meaning "childbirth" and the other meaning "pain in labour". It is possible to have either, they say, but it is not *necessary* to have the second.

Many women assume that childbirth will be painful. But using positive visualizations, such as imagining your body as a rose or lotus flower, or visiting your "safe place" (see box, p.29), combined with a supportive atmosphere, can transform birth from an experience of anxiety and tension into one of joy.

In seventeenth-century France, women kept a lighted candle and a "Rose of Jericho", or Resurrection Flower, by their bedside during labour. This "rose" is actually a desert plant that forms a tight ball when dry and unfolds and blooms when moistened. According to Christian folklore the flower was said to bloom at Christmas, close its petals on the anniversary of the Crucifixion and re-open them on the anniversary of the Resurrection. The unfolding flower is a symbolic reminder of the body opening for birth. The melting candle represents the progress of labour.

However, traditional birth aids are not always so poetic: the Rajputs (an Indian warrior caste) place a sickle, knife and plough-share beneath the bed to "cut" the pain. During a difficult labour, an African Ga midwife will give the mother a thorough brushing with a broom to chase away spirits.

Massage can be a wonderful birth tonic. In Bangladesh, massage by the *dai*, or midwife, is considered to be the best form of pain relief, as it provides constant physical and emotional support. During labour an Australian Aboriginal woman walks around, and leans against a tree. As birth approaches a female relative sits behind her and supports her back,

According to the Cuna Indians of Panama, a goddess, Muu, lives in the womb. During a difficult birth she is said to have become too attached to the baby and a special chanter is summoned to make her release the child.

while others massage her abdomen "to help the baby come down". To revive sluggish contractions, ask your birth assistant to massage the tops and soles of your feet, applying particular pressure to the heel and ankle (acupressure points); backache can be relieved with gentle circular massage.

In the Philippines, a midwife of the Bagos tribe performs the ritual of *kistat* – making as much noise as possible to force the baby out. In England, the pealing of church bells was believed to help delivery – perhaps the background noise made mothers feel less inhibited about shouting out. You could help banish your own inhibitions by preparing background music for birth. Experiment with a variety of moods to suit the changing emotions of labour. Gentle classical music, sounds of the rainforest and echoes of the sea can help you to focus in the early stages. African drumbeats and strong rhythms are wonderful at later active moments. Be sure to have some soft music ready to welcome your baby.

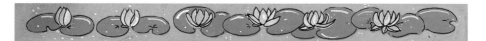

This way, that way, forwards and backwards

Take a tip from African women, who walk around for as long as possible during labour. "Active birth" means responding to your own body: dancing, leaning and crouching can all be part of your repertoire. When it comes to the moment of birth, each culture has its preferred position. You may be asked to lie on your back in a hospital, but in some tribes this position is taboo and thought to restrict the baby's blood supply. Zinacanteco women of Mexico crouch over a specially-woven reed mat; Sudanese women hang onto a rope suspended from the ceiling; African women often kneel in an upright position. A helpful recent addition to the birth kit is the bean bag, which adapts itself to any position you may choose.

Becoming a Father

*I*n Western culture, it is easy for fathers to feel left out during pregnancy and childbirth. Traditional societies often create significant roles for men in recognition of their importance in the child's life.

In China, a man's dreams about pregnancy are believed to be just as significant as a woman's: to dream of walking over a bridge holding hands with his wife, is an omen that his wife soon will be pregnant. A Chinese father-to-be is expected to visit the shrine of the goddess of childbirth, Guan Yin, before the birth of a child. He prays for his wife's safe deliverance and a healthy baby. Hawaiian tradition teaches that the actions of both parents during pregnancy influence the unborn child's nature, and fathers must take special care to be industrious and honest.

For thousands of years, fathers were encouraged to stay away from the birthing room: the strong magic surrounding childbirth was said to weaken male potency. Traditionally, African fathers visited mother and child only after the baby's cord stump had fallen off, when the "pollution of birth" (see p.44) was said to have disappeared. In Brazil, a man's bows and arrows were removed from the birthplace in case they became bewitched and ineffective.

Western fathers who do not wish to attend their baby's birth may be reassured to know that delivery is often swifter in an all-female environment. Men who prefer to be absent from the birth are often assigned "labours" of their own, such as bringing hot water and towels. In Slovakia, expectant fathers were sent to get a mouthful of water from a place where three streams converged and carry it in their mouths back to the mother. In rural Ireland men had to draw buckets of water continuously from a well until the baby was born.

According to middle-European tradition, it is possible for a man to tell if he is a father simply by the colour of his nipples. Pink nipples mean no children; brown indicate fatherhood.

During difficult births fathers often have special roles to play. Stripping off his clothes, a Zulu man offers his wife herbal medicine from his penis sheath. Among the Gusii people of Kenya, difficult labour is often thought to be caused by the baby being stuck some distance from the opening. The midwife will instruct the father to dig up roots of a bush called *chinsaga*; the juice of these roots, which the woman chews and sucks, encourages the child to come out.

In the Sherpa community of the Himalaya, fathers attend their wives throughout labour. Mother and father are united in a joint effort. The woman leans back against her husband and he massages her belly between contractions. After the baby has been born, he takes on the task of welcoming guests and makes sure that the breastfeeding mother is not overwhelmed by too many visitors. A Hiuchol Indian father shows a solidarity beyond the call of duty – a string is tied around his testicles, which can be pulled by his wife during contractions, so that he can share in her pain.

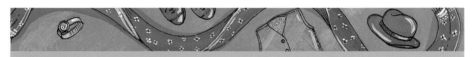

A Shared Experience

In the Yucatán, the baby's father is expected to be present during labour to "see how a woman suffers". The ancient tradition of couvade (from the Latin word *cubare*, meaning to lie down) requires a father to sympathize even more directly, by mirroring the experience of the mother in late pregnancy and childbirth. Before the birth the husband takes to his bed and fasts or abstains from certain foods. During his wife's labour the husband groans in simulated pain. Couvade is still practised today in South America, Siberia, Africa and Malaysia. Ritual clothes-swapping is a less demanding way of sharing childbirth. In remote parts of southern India, men don their wives' saris during childbirth. Traditionally, an Irish father gave symbolic strength to his wife in labour by giving her his waistcoat or watch to wear.

Honouring the Life Force

In Bangladesh the placenta is known as the "life force" and a baby is not considered to be fully alive until the placenta is laid out safely alongside him. However, in the West the placenta is commonly referred to as the "afterbirth", and is regarded as a mere inconvenience once the baby has emerged – most mothers never even see it.

Western doctors refer to the delivery of the placenta as the "third stage" of labour. A medically-managed third stage involves immediate clamping of the cord, separation of mother and baby, intramuscular drugs to produce contractions and a midwife to pull and push. However, left alone, the placenta may take half an hour to arrive, often after the mother has held the baby and put him to the breast; contact with the baby produces a rush of hormones which stimulate contractions and the placenta separates easily from the lining of the womb. In Africa the placenta is encouraged to emerge by means of a calabash (a seed gourd): the mother blows into the gourd and is also made to sneeze with pepper.

Once it has emerged, the placenta is subject to many different fates. Although it is true that in some cultures mothers cook and eat the placenta to give them strength, many people dwell on the spiritual significance of the "life force" rather than its nutritional value. The placenta's nurturing role in the womb is often believed to continue magically after birth and consequently it is treated with great reverence. In many cultures the placenta is buried beneath or near the house so that it is close to the baby. In ancient Egypt a pharaoh's placenta became one of the royal standards displayed on temple walls and carried on a pole in a leather bag during processions.

Balinese parents offer prayers for the *kanda empat*, or four siblings of the baby: placenta, amniotic fluid, blood and vernix. The four siblings are said to stand guard over the child in the womb and retain spiritual

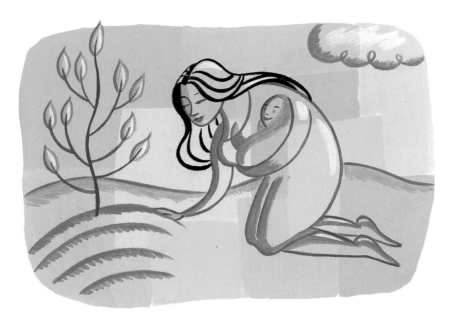

powers throughout a person's life; they are formally addressed at every important ceremony such as birthdays and weddings. The placenta is carefully washed and placed in a carved coconut shell and buried by the parents' front door.

The belief that a person's fate is intimately connected to the afterbirth is widespread. In Africa, where the baby's cord is cut with a reed, the placenta, cord and reed are kept by the mother and later buried in secrecy. The place of burial is the child's spiritual home. The Minangkabau of Sumatra say that a wandering child will always return home if his placenta is laid under the doorstep. However, if parents want their child to travel and seek his fortune, the placenta is thrown into the river. Among Tzotzil Indians in Mexico, if the baby is a boy, his father ties the cord to a high branch of a tree so that the child will be a fearless climber; a girl's cord is buried beneath the hearth to ensure that she will be a good helper to her mother.

If you decide to honour your baby's "life force" with a ceremonial burial, you could mark the spot with a special birth tree (see box, p.61).

Welcome to the World

In celebrating birth, we embrace the limitless possibilities of a new life. In nearly all cultures, traditions and rituals have emerged that, quietly or with fanfare, offer thanks for a safe delivery and welcome the baby into the world.

Large meals, often involving the whole community, are a common way to welcome a new baby. You may prefer to have a private session of thanksgiving after birth, and a party for family and friends a few weeks later when you feel stronger.

After a traditional European christening ceremony, alcohol is consumed, often in copious quantities, to "wet the baby's head". In Holland, the customary christening meal was very elaborate, with songs, speeches and a table laden with sugary delicacies. The *kandeel pot*, a tall goblet filled with sweetened Rhine wine, stood in the centre of the table and was stirred with a cinnamon stick – long for a boy, short for a girl.

In Brazil a Tapirape father colours his hair with red dye from the annatto tree to announce the arrival of his newborn child.

The element of water has always been connected with birth rites. The Christian tradition of baptism is intended to cleanse the baby from sin, and anointing the baby's head with blessed water originated with the early Indo-Europeans and is still practised by Hindu priests in India. On the morning of a Russian Orthodox christening, three days after the birth, the family collects "holy water" from a nearby river and sprinkles it around the house. At the christening feast the midwife serves a special porridge and is thanked for her services with coins from all the family, while the infant is presented with "teething" gifts.

The elements of fire and earth also play a part in traditional welcoming ceremonies. You could light a birth candle and pass the baby high over it, from mother to father, as is the custom in parts of Africa. In ancient Gaelic culture, a new baby would "take a turn through the smoke" soon after birth to drive away the Hidden People who were believed to cause harm by touching or singing to babies. The infant was handed back and forth three times, from midwife to father, across a candle flame. The midwife said a blessing (see p.50) and then the father carried his child three times around the flame. Or you could lay your baby to the ground in thanks to Mother Earth, as in ancient Rome. When the Roman father picked up his baby from the ground, it meant that he accepted paternity.

After the first intense weeks have passed, babies are often officially introduced to the outside world. A Guatemalan mother introduces her baby to nature when it is considered safe to take the child outside: she buries the umbilical cord in the earth, and visits streams, volcanos and trees with her baby asking for their protection in the child's future. You could create a similar ritual: take your baby to a park and carry her beneath the trees. Quietly, or in your head, ask the trees for their protection.

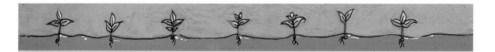

Planting a Birth Tree

For early civilizations, trees were the children who grew between Mother Earth and Father Sky, with their roots in the ground and their branches reaching heavenward. All over the world people plant trees to celebrate their offspring's arrival.

In Germany, fruit and nut trees are planted as symbolic companions for "the fruit of the womb" (the German word for fruit is *obst*, etymologically linked to "obstetrics"). In Nigeria, at the edge of every Ibo village is a banana grove. Each tree is named after the child for whom it was planted and the plantation serves as the village playground.

If you decide to plant a birth tree for your baby, you could plant an ash for long life, a fig for wisdom or an olive for peace. A maple tree is traditionally said to bring good luck.

The Gift of a Lifetime

In English folklore butterflies were said to be the souls of babies who had not yet been named. The act of naming a child is believed to be a covenant that binds the newborn child to the real world – now he is no longer a stranger but a member of a family and a wider community.

The time of naming varies greatly. In Christian cultures, where a name was traditionally regarded as an important form of spiritual protection, naming ceremonies take place very soon after birth. However, in the Nicobar Islands in the Indian Ocean, names are given as a sign of independence and are only bestowed when a child begins to walk.

In many cultures a name is regarded as a significant gift to the child rather than as a means of identification: parental choices are replete with meaning, whether spiritual, social or shrewdly descriptive. For the Ibani of Nigeria the name Bitegeriagha, "a cloth cannot speak", expresses the inherent value of the child (cloth is the Ibani measure of wealth).

Children are often named according to parents' hopes and expectations. A boy from Vietnam might be called Tuan Ahn, meaning Famous One. An Arab girl could be Saideh (Lucky).

Possibly the most uninspired way to name a child is by order of birth, but in the days of large families this was not uncommon. Many boys in ancient Rome were called simply Primus, Secundus, Tertius (First, Second, Third) – or Prima, Secunda, Tertia for girls. Balinese parents start with a number-name, but then elaborate it as they get to know the child. A fourth-born who was easily upset became Ketut Jangling – "fourth child who cries when he is put down".

Although in the West names come in and out of fashion, there is often a generational cycle, with grandparents and babies sharing the same name. According to traditional Jewish custom, children are named after loved ones who have died, thus creating a name chain that can be traced right back through the family tree.

"A good name is better than precious ointment."

Ecclesiastes 7:1

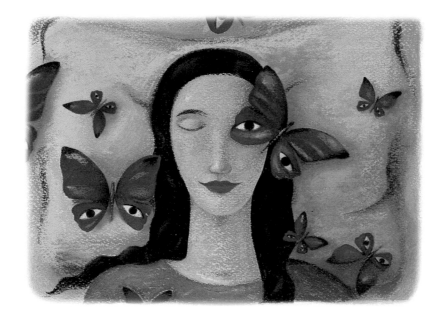

If you are having difficulty choosing the right name, try the Hawaiian method of dreaming the answer. Before sleeping, meditate on your baby, and ask yourself to dream of a name. It might be spoken, or revealed symbolically for you to interpret: dreaming of a princess could imply the Hebrew name Sarah (which itself means "princess"). If you dream of a king, you might choose the royal Scottish name Duncan, or the Jewish Saul, according to your own tradition. Flower-names such as Rose or Lily might spring from the unconscious mind, while a dream about rocks or mountains might lead you to Peter, which is derived from the Greek word *petras*, meaning "rock", or Winston, which means "friendly rock".

A name given at birth is not always permanent. In many cultures individuals take on new names as they grow older and their appearance changes or their character becomes more evident. For example, the African name Masani means "child who has a gap between the teeth" (a portent of good luck), is obviously given after teeth appear.

The Path of Destiny

A new baby is a mystery: who will she become? In the face of life's uncertainties people have devised many systems of predicting and explaining a child's destiny.

The time of birth has always played a pivotal role in systems of fate and prediction. In the Scottish Highlands, certain days of the week are considered to be more auspicious than others: Tuesday's child will be "solemn and sad", while Wednesday's is "merry and glad". (Watch out for Thursday's child who is supposed to be "inclined to thieving"!) In Christian tradition a child is believed to be especially blessed if born on a Sunday. German mothers said that the Sabbath child grows up strong and beautiful, while Scandinavians believed that Sunday's children could see spirits.

Filipino babies born at night are said to be braver than those born during the day. In Welsh folklore, the infant born at sunrise is destined to be intelligent and successful, while the baby who emerges at sunset is inclined to be lazy and lacking in ambition. Traditional English custom, meanwhile, holds that children born at the hours of three, six, nine and twelve – when church bells traditionally chimed – will have the gift of prophecy, or "second sight", and an immunity to witchcraft. To be born during the incoming tide, a harbinger of new life, is often thought to be lucky in coastal regions.

Ga women in western Africa say that the pregnant woman's environment shapes the temperament of her child. If she lives on plains of burnt grass, her child will be smooth-skinned and very dark. If she lives on a hill with distant views, her child will be tall, healthy and strong. Should she live near the sea, her children will be as lively and loud as the crashing surf.

Many cultures have looked to the stars to reveal individual destiny. The position of the sun in the stars at the time of birth gives the child's zodiac sign and each sign is believed to carry certain personality traits (see p.66).

In places where the weather changes swiftly, the type of conditions prevailing at the time of birth are said to affect the personality of the baby. In parts of the Philippines, it is said that children born in a rainstorm will be troublesome, while a child born on a sunny day will always be full of joy.

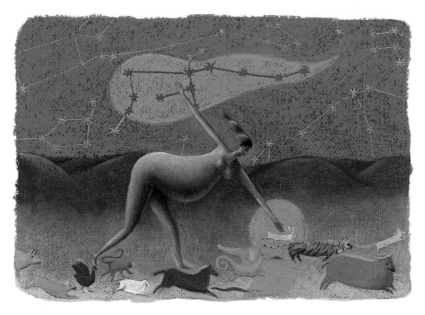

Western astrologers also predict the patterns of a child's life by drawing up a "horoscope" – a chart showing the relative positions of the sun, moon, stars and planets with respect to the exact time and place of a person's birth. The horoscope will identify the heavenly influences at work throughout the child's life. Its interpretation will show the course that his life might take, including the kind of work to which he might be best suited; his relationships with other family members; or the zodiac sign of his ideal future partner.

The Chinese zodiac (see p.67) is based on a cyclical twelve-year system, which aligns each personality with a particular animal. In Chinese legend, the twelve animals quarrelled about who should be first in the cycle. The gods held a contest – whoever could reach the opposite riverbank first would have that privilege. As the animals jumped in the river, the Rat climbed onto the Ox's back. The Ox looked set to win, but just before he reached the bank, the Rat leapt ashore before him and so won the race. The Pig, who was the laziest, came last.

The Western Zodiac

Aries, *The Ram*
March 21 – April 19
Full of energy and enthusiasm, these children make great leaders.

Taurus, *The Bull*
April 20 – May 20
Cautious but practical children who are loyal to their friends.

Gemini, *The Twins*
May 21 – June 21
Bright, witty personalities who are apt to be fidgety, or chatterboxes.

Libra, *The Scales*
September 23 – October 23
Harmonious children who love their friends, but can be a little lazy.

Scorpio, *The Scorpion*
October 24 – November 21
*Powerful personalities who enjoy puzzles and mysteries –
they are rarely ill.*

Sagittarius, *The Archer*
November 22 – December 21
*Sagittarius children have great insight and demand to
be treated fairly.*

Cancer, *The Crab*
June 22 – July 22
Sensitive and emotional children who like to care for others.

Leo, *The Lion*
July 23 – August 22
*Like to be the centre of attention, but they are also
loving and generous.*

Virgo, *The Maiden*
August 23 – September 22
Often perfectionist, these children have keen analytical minds.

Capricorn, *The Goat*
December 22 – January 19
Practical, serious children with ambition and drive.

Aquarius, *The Water Carrier*
January 20 – February 18
These children love anything new or different – they are easily bored.

Pisces, *The Fish*
February 19 – March 20
*Extremely inventive, sensitive children who need quiet times
to themselves.*

The Chinese Zodiac

Years of the Rat (1984, 1996, 2008)
Rats are charming and ambitious.

Years of the Ox (1985, 1997, 2009)
Oxen are patient and confident.

Years of the Tiger (1986, 1998, 2010)
Tigers are sensitive and courageous.

Years of the Rabbit (1987, 1999, 2011)
Rabbits are articulate and clever.

Years of the Dragon (1988, 2000, 2012)
Dragons are energetic and soft-hearted.

Years of the Snake (1989, 2001, 2013)
Snakes are wise and intense.

Years of the Horse (1990, 2002, 2014)
Horses are popular and perceptive.

Years of the Sheep (1991, 2003, 2015)
Sheep are elegant and gentle.

Years of the Monkey (1992, 2004, 2016)
Monkeys are inventive and flexible.

Years of the Rooster (1993, 2005, 2017)
Roosters are capable and solitary.

Years of the Dog (1994, 2006, 2018)
Dogs are loyal and honest.

Years of the Pig (1995, 2007, 2019)
Pigs are studious and kind.

Birthstones

- *January* – Garnet (dark red)
- *February* – Amethyst (purple)
- *March* – Aquamarine (pale blue)
- *April* – Diamond (white/clear)
- *May* – Emerald (bright green)
- *June* – Pearl/Moonstone (creamy white)
- *July* – Ruby (red)
- *August* – Peridot (pale green)
- *September* – Sapphire (deep blue)
- *October* – Opal/Rose Zircon (pale pink)
- *November* – Golden Topaz/Citrine (yellow)
- *December* – Turquoise/Blue Topaz (sky blue)

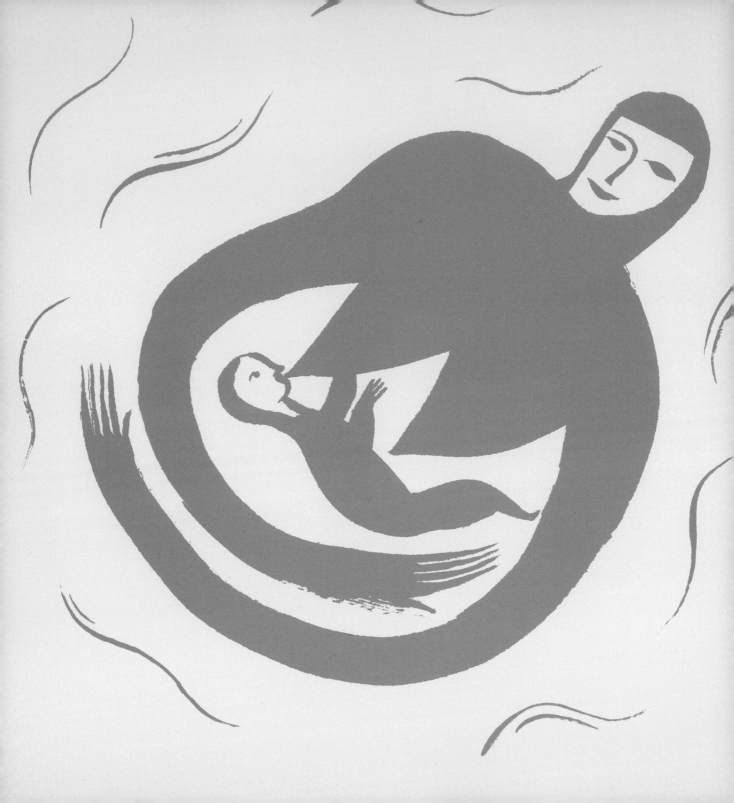

Early Days

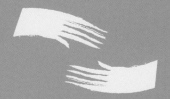

A baby is a question mark and his mother the answer he seeks. Sensitive to every new encounter, the newborn experiences life through the soft filter of mother's embrace, her milk, her lullabies. He recognizes you by sight and by touch – you sense his needs and his separate self.

Together, you will learn.

An Instinctive Connection

Some people say that there's no such thing as maternal instinct – for them the mysterious act of mothering is simply a bundle of skills that can be learned on the job – by anyone.

Of course, if we spend enough time with a baby, we may anticipate her needs – given the right care and attention, from various sources, a baby will thrive. Yet biological and anthropological evidence (and common sense) support the idea that mothers are specifically suited to care for their own offspring. Women's bodies have evolved to accommodate the nine-month incubation of babies and their milk is adapted for long-term breast-feeding. These functions suggest that nature intended for mothers and babies to spend their time together, and in most societies, they do.

Mothering skills are not indelible, however: they can be honed or lost. For example, few Western women know when their babies want to urinate, yet many babies around the world do not wear diapers or nappies. Instead, mothers hold the baby at arm's length. When a Netsilik woman was asked how she knew when to do this, she replied: "How could any mother be so dumb not to know?" Many aspects of motherhood do not need to be taught. Studies show that pregnant women predict the weight of their babies more accurately than doctors or machines. First-time mothers put infants to the breast without the need for demonstration and rock their babies at sixty to seventy beats a minute, similar to the rhythm of the adult's heart; they also tend to carry infants on their left-hand side – near the maternal heartbeat. New mothers can often recognize the sound of their own infant in a ward of crying babies, and most mothers can recognize the unique scent of their babies.

"There is no such thing as a baby, there is a baby and someone."

D. W. Winnicott
(20th-century British psychoanalyst)

Besides the instinctive physical triggers, there are more mysterious aspects. Some mothers have a "sixth sense" when their children are in danger. They seem to have telepathic conversations and early-warning signs if their baby is becoming unwell – these are scientifically inexplicable. An intact maternal instinct surrounds a child like an aura, protecting her in countless subtle ways.

Many mothers expect to feel an immediate bond with their new baby and become anxious if instead they feel rather detached. For some, the connection begins before birth – a dream or an event may suddenly intensify feelings for the baby. But others do not feel instant adoration, even when the baby is finally in their arms. Of course, there are those who fall in love at first sight, but bonding is an intangible, highly personal process, and slow bonding is normal too.

Everyday acts of caring such as soothing your little one to sleep, or holding her to your breast, create the ties that bind you for ever.

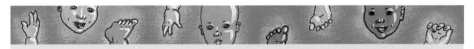

A Mother-and-Baby Honeymoon

We usually think of a honeymoon as a time of privacy for a husband and wife but, in many cultures, the tradition of undisturbed intimacy applies also to a mother and her baby immediately after the birth. The Wayãpo tribe of Brazil observe a "moon-long" seclusion for a newly delivered mother and child, during which time they bond with one another and learn each other's shapes and smells.

In India, according to ancient Ayurvedic principles, new mothers are looked after in their homes for the first twenty-two days after the birth. During this period, the mother-infant bond develops as the mother remains focused only on nurturing, holding, stroking and generally getting to know her baby. Breastfeeding develops smoothly and naturally, free from any pressure to clock-watch.

Mothering the Mother

The first weeks after birth are an important time for a mother and baby. As well as being the honeymoon period (see box, p.71), this is a particularly crucial time for the mother in which to rest and recuperate. A new mother needs to be reassured and nurtured almost as much as her newborn baby.

In many cultures a new mother is exempt from her normal duties and is looked after by a team of family and friends. Special meals prepared for postnatal women are chosen for their special strength-giving properties. Sudanese women are brought daily gifts of goat's or camel's milk; in India, family members prepare nourishing lentil soups, and a concoction of nuts, raisins, lotus seeds and ghee is stored ready for the seclusion period. In Switzerland, newly delivered mothers were brought the first pickings from cherry trees – apart from being a delicious treat, this practice was thought to ensure a good cherry crop.

A traditional midwife often stays during the "honeymoon", to teach the mother about babycare and provide her with healing baths and soothing massages. Ilocanos mothers in the Philippines are given a ritual bath in *a-nger* (boiled guava leaves) and regular abdominal massages. You may like to try a sitz bath with a few drops each of cypress and lavender essential oils, both of which aid healing and protect against infection. Moroccan mothers are massaged with henna, walnut bark and kohl; traditional Hawaiian midwives give a vigorous circular *lomi-lomi* massage with their fingers, elbows and thumbs; and in western India, the midwife-maid massages the mother with coconut oil.

Japanese women wear a *hari-obi* ("wide sash") in pregnancy to support the abdomen; they also wear it for about three weeks after birth to help them get back into shape. To make your own use a piece of cloth 8in (20 cm) by 6ft, 6in (2m), wrapped three or

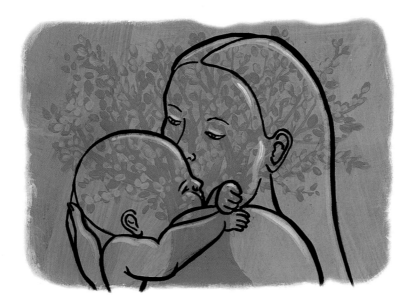

four times around your lower back and stomach. Take care not to bind it too tightly – the idea is to support the uterus, not restrict circulation.

In some cultures this time of rest and recuperation is strictly imposed and surrounded by taboos aimed at protecting the new mother and baby from evil spirits and society from the perceived "pollution" (see p.44) associated with childbirth. Only after several days is the mother received back into the wider community, often with a symbolic purification ritual. In Jewish law, a mother is considered *nidoh* ("impure") for seven days after

the birth of a boy and four days after a girl. After seven subsequent "clean" days she is ritually immersed in purifying water. Meanwhile, in European Christian tradition, women were "churched" a few weeks after childbirth. This process (a medieval ritual once practised all over the Christian world) was, in effect, a church service to welcome a new mother back into the heart of the community after her period of seclusion. She would return to society refreshed and relaxed, ready to show off her beautiful new baby – already secure in and trustful of his mother's arms.

Nature's Vaccine

Most people recognize the benefits of mother's milk, but what about the honey that comes first? The value of colostrum, "nature's vaccine", has been neglected for centuries.

This rich pre-milk is produced in late pregnancy and for three days after birth. It is nearly invisible – occasionally you may see a golden droplet on the nipple – but many mothers simply have to trust that they are producing it. Perhaps its visual insignificance is the reason why some cultures are happy to ignore it, but others go further, banning colostrum with strong taboos.

The sooner a baby begins suckling, the better: for a few hours after birth, colostrum contains enormous quantities of antibodies. On the first day it teems with fatty acids, growth factors, vitamins, zinc, immune defences and anti-infectious properties. Colostrum is particularly rich in vitamin A to supplement the low liver reserves of newborns. However, this potency is short-lived: as breastmilk replaces colostrum, protective cells decrease from millions to thousands. The Gusii tribe of Kenya nurse their babies from the first day and value the colostrum, which, they say, "makes the child fat".

Evolution designed babies to be put straight to the breast, but in many places the demands of religion and medical theory cause the remarkable benefits of colostrum to be lost. In Bangladesh, colostrum is known as "bad milk". Newborn babies are given honey and cow's milk, or mustard oil diluted in pond water, until the mother begins to produce milk. More than 2,000 years ago, Ayurvedic doctors insisted that new babies were fed honey and clarified butter until breastmilk began to flow. Breton mothers in France have a tradition of not feeding their babies before baptism, which usually takes place when the baby is three days old, and the valuable colostrum is ignored. In Japan, babies were fed *jumigokoto*, an

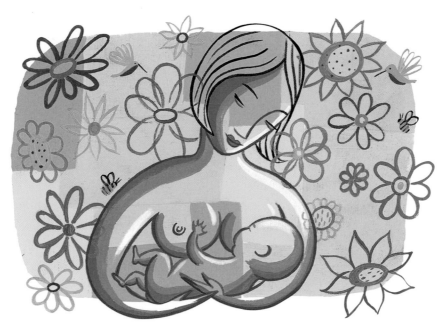

elixir of roots and herbs, until the mother's milk arrived. Some southern African tribes begin feeding their off-spring on a diet of watery porridge rather than the perfectly packaged liquid meals a mother can provide.

Apart from the physical benefits to the new baby, the mother also profits psychologically by breastfeeding her baby from the outset. Successful breastfeeding often begins in the "practice" days before milk begins to flow and breasts become full: neglect of the colostrum days may result in a loss of confidence and cause difficulty with breastfeeding later on.

Some mothers are encouraged to bottlefeed a new baby in order to maintain high blood sugar levels. However, it is perfectly normal for a newborn to have low blood sugar for some hours after the birth – frequent breastfeeding soon improves the balance. Keep your baby near you with plenty of skin-to-skin contact. This will stimulate the "colostrum ejection reflex". Try to limit the number of visitors you receive at this important time. Concentrate for now upon each other, and your baby will think that he has arrived in a land of milk and honey.

A Mother's Milk

Breastfeeding is not just a form of nourishment – it is also a powerful and subtle form of communication, enhanced by stroking, playfulness and eye-contact. For your baby, it is a wonderful feast, engaging all her senses. A mother's natural food supply is also nutritionally ideal for the newborn.

Even in societies where babies are denied the breast for the first three days (for various reasons), mothers may go on to nurse until the child is two or three years old – or even older. While solids are also gradually introduced, breastfeeding provides an emotional continuum, a reassuring point of contact for both a mother and her baby.

Women among the !Kung hunter-gatherers of Botswana and Namibia follow a common breastfeeding pattern that was probably known to the earliest humans – and it works to the mutual benefit of baby and mother.

Babies suckle briefly and often throughout the day and night, creating a perfect rhythm of supply and demand. Breastfeeding problems are extremely rare. Contraception is unknown, but the baby's suckling stimulates production of the breastfeeding hormone prolactin, which also suppresses ovulation. Hence, the frequent nursing helps to ensure a gap of up to four years between each child.

Although we may not be able to offer our babies the same level of skin-to-skin contact, we can learn from societies where breastfeeding is assumed to be normal. Difficult or uncomfortable breastfeeding is often the result of insufficient feeds or poor positioning of the baby (with gums on the nipple, rather than over the areola). Problems with breastfeeding occur mainly in cultures where mothers rarely see each other nursing. Girls who witness breastfeeding on a daily basis absorb the techniques unconsciously from an early age.

One of the keys to breastfeeding is the simple knowledge that every woman can do it. You need no equipment nor any special attributes. One useful piece of information to aid trouble-free breastfeeding is that the nipples are best left unwashed – soap spoils the natural aroma of your skin to which your baby is attuned. Washing with soap also reduces the moisture of the areola.

If problems do occur, there are countless traditional remedies. Mothers in southeast Asia believe that they can increase their milk supply by eating the flowers of a banana tree and nourishing chicken broth. To prevent their nipples from becoming dry, Taralpe women of Brazil moisturize them with honey; alternatively, the Magar of Nepal use apricot oil. If your breasts become engorged (too full), try the old European remedy of cabbage leaves, with holes cut for the nipples. Apply cold, raw leaves after each feed (they will fit snugly inside a bra), and leave them against your breasts until the leaves have reached room temperature. Cracked nipples respond to a treatment that couldn't be easier to find – moisturize them with a few drops of breastmilk.

The Birth of the Milky Way

According to Greek legend, the hero Heracles was born to the mortal Alcmene, as a result of her secret liaison with the god Zeus. After his labours on earth, Heracles ascended to Olympus to become an Immortal. He was "reborn" to Hera, goddess of marriage and maternity, in an adoption ritual once practised by barbarian tribes. Hera went to bed in mock labour and "produced" baby Heracles from under the sheets. However, having been born originally to a mortal mother, Heracles had yet to achieve true immortality. Zeus placed him secretly in Hera's bed to suckle her divine milk. Unaware of his strength, Heracles sucked so eagerly that Hera's milk spilled across the night sky, creating the phenomenon we know as the Milky Way.

Sleep, Baby, Sleep

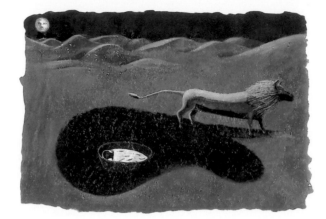

In Central America, each newborn baby has a nahual *or animal twin, which protects him during sleep. To discover the beast's identity, a circle of ashes is placed around the baby's sleeping place, in which the* nahual *leaves tell-tale footprints. A taboo is proclaimed against killing the beast and, in return, the* nahual *becomes the child's lifelong protector.*

By night as by day, traditional societies ensure magical protection for their babies. Nightmares are particularly frightening for children and have been widely believed to be caused by malevolent spirits. In ancient Greece, parents would spend a night with their baby in the temple of Hypnos (the god of sleep) to be sure of the god's protection against night-time visitations by evil spirits. In Eastern Europe, mothers would place a small broom under a baby's pillow, to sweep away evil spirits; and Romanies tucked sprigs of rosemary under the pillow to ensure sweet dreams. According to an old English tradition, moving the child's bed from a north-south to an east-west position was also said to prevent disturbed sleep. English cradles were often made from ash wood, which was believed to have protective qualities.

Feng Shui for the Sleeping Place

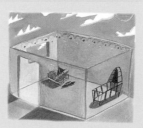

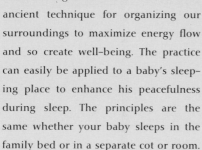

The Chinese believe that energy (*qi*) flows through everything around us. When this energy becomes blocked, we feel unease. Feng Shui is the ancient technique for organizing our surroundings to maximize energy flow and so create well–being. The practice can easily be applied to a baby's sleeping place to enhance his peacefulness during sleep. The principles are the same whether your baby sleeps in the family bed or in a separate cot or room.

The door of a baby's bedroom should always be left open to allow energy to flow easily into and out of the room. However, the cradle, cot or family bed should never be placed in the direct line of incoming energy (directly opposite the door), as this is said to disturb the baby's sleep. Try positioning your baby's sleeping place against a wall with the doorway in sight, so that he can see whoever is coming into the room. Avoid placing a baby's bed beneath a window, as the passage from door to window is an energy highway, which could cause interruption to your baby's restful sleep.

According to the principles of Feng Shui, the walls of a baby's bedroom should be decorated predominantly in the colour associated with the baby's Chinese birth element. For example, if your baby is born into the wood element, the room should be blue; into fire, green; into earth, red; into metal, yellow; and into water, white. You could decorate the room with pictures of your baby's Chinese birth animal (see p.67).

If there is a mirror in the room, be sure not to place it opposite the foot of the cradle or bed, or directly opposite the door. Positive energy travelling through the room will be reflected off the glass and back onto a resting baby, and this may disrupt his peaceful sleep.

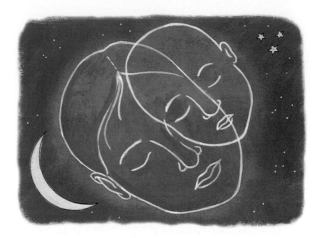

As they grow, children of many cultures are encouraged to share their beds with their siblings or other family members for safety and warmth. In the Dani tribe of Irian Jaya, men and boys sleep together on large mats and wake often during the night. They tell a story or stoke the fire and then doze off again.

Many traditions imply that the baby has his own sleeping place – a crib in the parent's room or, as in most modern Western homes, in a different room altogether. However, there are a significant number of cultures in which a new-born baby is brought into the parental bed to sleep beside his mother, where her familiar presence, the warmth of her body, her smell and her caresses all help the baby to sleep easily, as he did in the womb. Infant sleep disturbance and adult insomnia are rare in places where parents and babies "co-sleep". Throughout Asia, Africa, South America and among certain tribes in Australasia and North America, co-sleeping is a way of life: babies sleep with their mother in hammocks or on mats made of bamboo, bark, rags or leaves.

Many parents fear that they would roll on top of their infant during the night, but studies have shown that, even during sleep, parents are acutely aware of their baby's presence. In order to create your own co-sleeping environment, your mattress must be firm and pillows should be kept away from the baby's head. Be very careful not to smoke or drink too much before welcoming your baby into the safety of your own bed.

Dreamcatching

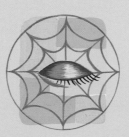

Dreamcatchers are hanging dream filters, traditionally made by Lakota Native Americans and suspended near the sleeping place. The dreamcatcher traps nightmares within its web and allows smooth, sweet dreams to pass through.

Dreamcatchers may be bought but a homemade one can be more personal. To make a traditional dreamcatcher (as wide as an average adult hand), you will need approximately 4ft (1.2m) of soaked willow bough (or grapevine) and 10ft (3m) of strong, thin string. Bend the willow to create a hoop of double thickness, and bind it where the ends meet.

A dreamcatcher is made using one stitch over and over again. Tie the string onto the hoop, leaving a short loose end to make a loop for hanging (call this point on the hoop twelve o'clock). Take the long end of the string and (not too tightly) stretch the string across the hoop to two o'clock. Pass the string around the back of the willow and up through the hole between string and hoop, making a knot which will anchor this point. Pull the stitch taut but not tight. Continue around the hoop, making stitches at four, six, eight and ten o'clock. For the second and subsequent rounds, make the stitches around the previous round of string. As you pull gently, the stitches form diamond shapes and a web will appear.

On the third round, add a bead to represent the spider in the web. When the stitches become too small to pass the string through, leave a hole in the centre and finish with a knot, allowing 6–8in (15–20cm) of string to tie on two or three feathers. The dreamcatcher should reflect the person it protects – attach thread from your baby's scarf or a favourite teddy's ribbon. Beads and feathers added at a new moon increase the magic. Early morning rays cleanse the dreamcatcher for another night.

Rock-A-Bye Baby

Sung by mothers and nurses all over the world to coax babies to sleep, lullabies use the soft hum and gentle rhythm of simple tunes and phrases to re-create for the baby a sense that she is safe in the womb. Combined with gentle rocking, lullabies give the reassuring message: drift off to sleep, mother is here, all is well with the world.

Russia

Sleep, ah sleep, my darling baby,
Su, su, lullaby.
See the moon is watching o'er thee,
Peacefully on high.
Thou shalt hear a wondrous story,
Close each wakeful eye,
And a song as well I'll sing thee,
Su, su, lullaby.

England

Sweet and low, sweet and low,
Wind of the western sea.
Low, low, breathe and blow –
Wind of the western sea!
Over the rolling waters go;
Come from the dying moon and blow,
Blow him again to me;
While my little one, while my pretty
   one, sleeps.

Creole

Go to sleep, Colas little Brother,
Go to sleep, sweet dreams be with you.
Mamma will bake a sweet little cake,
Papa's here with choc'late for you.
Go to sleep, Colas little brother
Go to sleep, sweet dreams be with you.

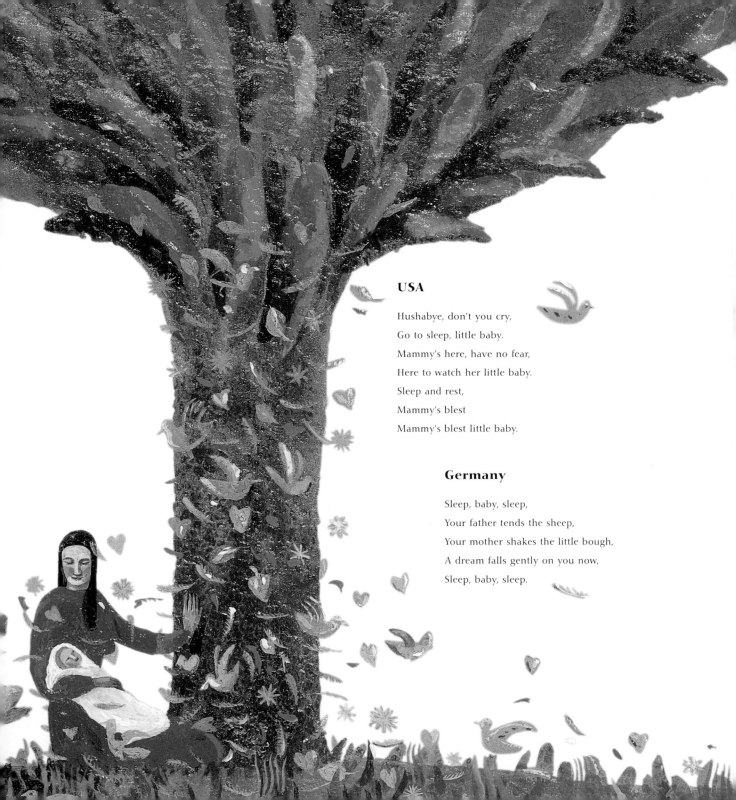

USA

Hushabye, don't you cry,
Go to sleep, little baby.
Mammy's here, have no fear,
Here to watch her little baby.
Sleep and rest,
Mammy's blest
Mammy's blest little baby.

Germany

Sleep, baby, sleep,
Your father tends the sheep,
Your mother shakes the little bough,
A dream falls gently on you now,
Sleep, baby, sleep.

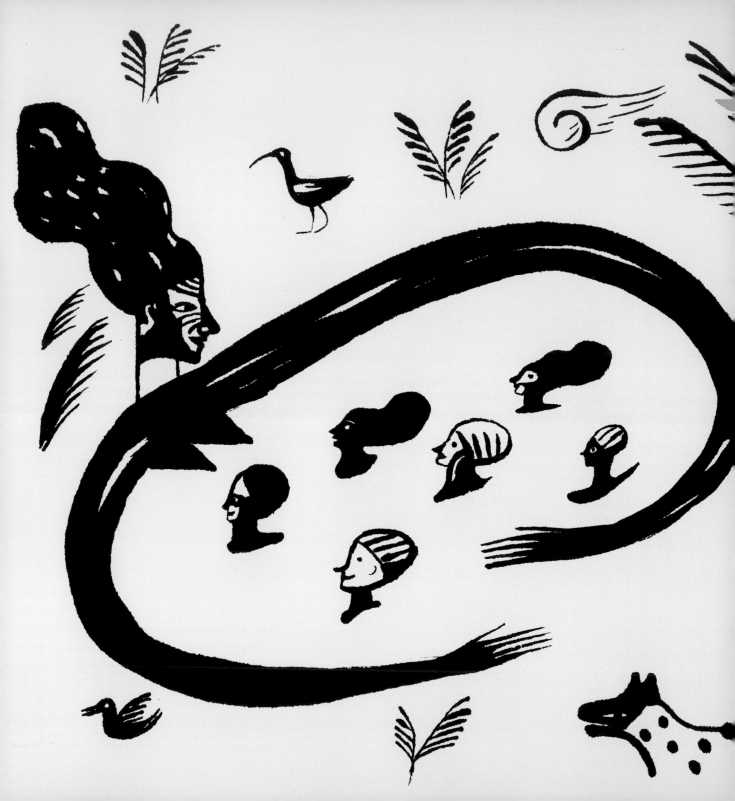

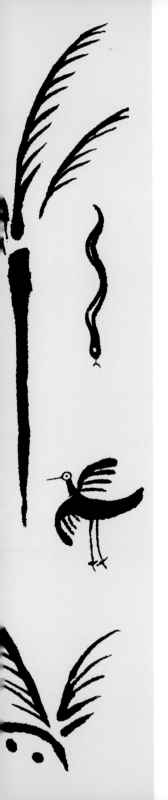

Everything Came from Her

"My early years are connected ... with my mother. ... I can remember the comforting feel of her body as she carried me on her back. ... When I was hungry or thirsty she would swing me round to where I could reach her full breasts. ... At night when there was no sun to warm me, her arms, her body took its place; and as I grew older ... from my safe place on her back I could watch without fear as I wanted, and when sleep overcame me I had only to close my eyes."

Kabongo, an East–African
Kikiyu chief, remembers
his early years

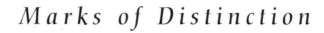

Marks of Distinction

*B*eing born "in the caul", with the amniotic sac still intact around the baby, or with part of it attached to the baby's head, has been considered a good omen since at least Roman times. In France, a person who is persistently lucky is said to have been *né coiffé* (literally "born in the veil"). Cauls were widely believed to have protective qualities, which could be transferred to a new owner if the caul changed hands. Sailors (among others) paid high prices for cauls, which were believed to protect against drowning. In Jewish tradition, a caul was believed to shield the owner from storm demons.

There are many other marks of distinction apparent at birth that have given rise to a variety of tradition and lore. The type of birthmark known as a strawberry mark first appears as a tiny red dot, which gradually swells in size to resemble the fruit of its name. In parts of England, these marks are said to be caused by the mother-to-be eating too many strawberries during pregnancy, while in rural America, they are said to be the result of a pregnant woman being denied her strawberry cravings. Alarming as they might seem, strawberry marks usually fade within a few years (most likely by the time the child is three or four).

In many cultures, for a pregnant woman to look at an eclipse is regarded as the cause of unusual body markings on her baby. In Mexico, if a pregnant woman witnesses a lunar eclipse her baby may have extra fingers or toes. Salmon-pink scratches on the baby's forehead, eyelids and neck are known in Europe as "stork bites", derived from the tradition that babies are carried in slings by storks. The marks were said to be accidentally caused while the bird carried the baby in a bundle, suspended from its beak. Also called "angel kisses", these marks are a collection of tiny blood vessels below the skin, which soon fade.

In Europe a birthmark was often believed to be caused by the pregnant

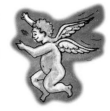

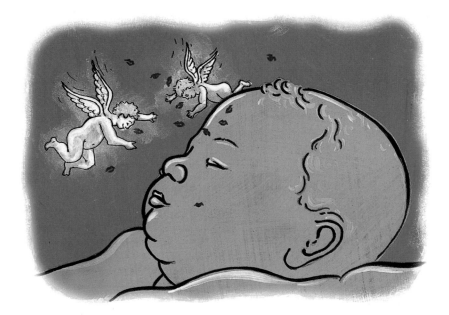

mother being frightened by something. The mark would sometimes represent the object of fear: the shape of a dog's tooth might mean that a dog caused a fright. Birthmarks were said to fade if licked by the mother.

A Cherokee father traditionally avoids denting his hat during his wife's pregnancy to avoid causing dents in the baby's head. However, all babies are born with a small gap, where their skull bones should meet, called a "fontanelle". It takes months, sometimes years, for the gap to harden over, and great care must be taken to protect the baby's head. In southern African tribes, evil spirits are said to enter through the fontanelle.

When an Anbarra Aboriginal baby is born, his parents look for a special mark to identify the child's totemic animal. This mark corresponds to the spot where the father speared an animal while hunting and then gave it to the mother. The animal's spirit entered the mother's uterus and the child's special mark is a visual sign of the continuing totem spirit (see p.20).

Protecting the Newborn

Newborn babies are universally believed to be vulnerable creatures – in many cultures the dangers are seen to be spiritual as well as physical. Protective charms are often considered as important as medicine and common sense to ensure the safety of a newborn baby.

In the Middle East and southern Asia newborns are believed to be especially vulnerable to the "evil eye", reflecting a widespread belief that spirits, and sometimes other people, are jealous of the new baby and can harm her with envious glances. Relatives are careful not to praise a child too enthusiastically in case they attract unwelcome attention; babies also wear amulets (often eye-shapes made of blue glass) to avert malevolent influences.

In European tradition, boys are dressed in blue, girls in pink. Blue, the sacred colour of the heavens, was traditionally used as a divine and magical shield for male infants. (Girls, who were less desirable to the evil spirits, wore pink, the colour of European skin.) Evidence of the belief in the magical power of blue is also found in the Middle East, where an entire household – including the new baby in it – was safeguarded by painting the front door a brilliant sky blue.

Among the Native American Hopi tribe, sacred corn ears are placed on either side of the baby's cradle for the first twenty days of her life. In ancient Rome, a nine-day-old baby was given a *bulla* – a rounded metal or leather box containing a charm to ward off evil spirits. The child would keep the *bulla* until she made the transition to adulthood at puberty.

In ancient Egypt, the cat goddess, Bastet, was the Nurse of Royal Children, but she came to be the guardian of all infants, seeing them safely through to adolescence. Amulets and talismans made from blue-green earthenware have been found, showing a cat with swollen teats surrounded by kittens. From 1000 to 500BCE, Bastet's cult was at its height, and during

"... to make you strong and fair and always young and to keep back death and sorrow, and to keep you safe from other winds and evil spirits."

An Irish woman's prayer as she holds up a new baby to the south wind

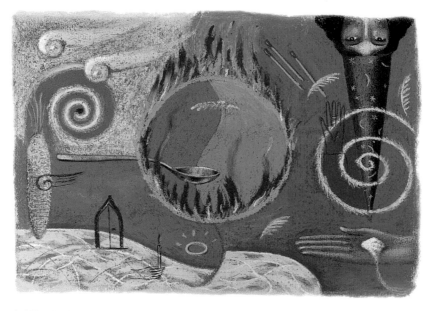

childbirth her image was worn on necklaces to safeguard both the mother and child. Once a baby had been born, a cat silhouette was often tattooed on her arm to ensure Bastet's lasting protection; some parents even went so far as to inject their babies with a few drops of blood from a sacred cat. Children were often named to ensure her guardianship – for example, *Djed-Bastet-iouef-ankh*, meaning "Bastet–said Let–him–live".

An *Ojo de Dios*, "God's Eye", was an ancient talisman made by the Huichol people of Mexico. You might like to try making one of your own. You need two straight twigs and various coloured yarns. Form a cross–shape with the sticks and, using some yarn, bind them with diagonal strokes in both directions across the centre. This is the "iris" of the *Ojo de Dios*, ready to protect your new baby. At each birthday, tie on a new colour, wrapping it around each spoke of the cross, to make a diamond shape. Every year a different coloured yarn is woven around the "eye", until the fifth birthday when the charm is complete, giving you a memento to treasure.

Forget-Me-Not

*A*fter giving birth, many women speak of a feeling that they somehow brushed with death. This is usually an emotion of quiet triumph over danger, yet every culture has to acknowledge the vulnerability of the mother and infant. When a baby does not survive his perilous journey into life, how can you begin to face the indescribable loss?

If a baby dies before birth, it is particularly hard to hold on to tangible memories. Miscarriage and stillbirth are underplayed in Western society, where parents expect every pregnancy to result in parenthood. But in Mexico they say that each star in the sky shines for a miscarried baby. In Japan there is a temple near Tokyo where thousands of parents have placed stone Buddhas in memory of their unborn children.

Inevitably, the risk of infant death varies dramatically according to the time and place of a baby's birth. One of the safest places to give birth is Holland, where careful screening means that low-risk pregnancies usually end in a home birth with little interference, while women at risk of complications can make the most of state-of-the-art equipment. But no country can guarantee a safe delivery – some things are beyond our control.

Twin births are generally more risky than single births. Among the Yoruba tribe in Nigeria, where many twins are born, wooden figurines are carved to represent each twin. If one should die, the twin doll is carried around, washed and dressed in memory of the lost child.

In northern Thailand, the Karen tribe believe that a child's own spirit decides how long to live and so parents should not be heartbroken when a baby dies, as this is his spirit's wish. It is said that death is easy for a tiny baby, sometimes easier than choosing life, although it can take parents many years to feel like choosing life again.

Some tribes believe that unborn and newborn babies are all essentially spirit children, whose hold on life is not strong; if they die, their souls fly back to the spirit world to make a new start. A Malay baby who dies before he is five months old still shares his mother's soul. However comforting this image may be, parents still need to feel the physical closeness of a baby who is very ill or dying. It helps to hold him, to stroke his skin, to talk and share intimacies. We need to gather memories, however small. Photographs, the hospital

wristband, a flower that was pressed into the baby's hand, an item of clothing – mementos like these ensure that his life, however brief, will not be forgotten.

There are other ways in which to keep the memory alive and acknowledge your grief and loss. Planting a tree or a small garden for the child is a symbol of faith in new life. As it grows, so will your hope and recovery. Perhaps you need a special place where you can go to be with your memories. It might be an empty beach or a park full of children. Wherever you are, your baby will always be connected to you.

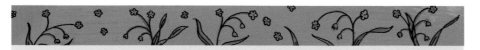

Memory and Hope

"**I** remember you in this solemn hour, my beloved child. I remember the days when I still delighted in your bloom, in your bodily and mental growth, in beautiful hopes for your future. The inscrutable will of God took you early from me; He called you to His abode; yet in my wounded heart the fond remembrance of you can never be extinguished. But the Almighty is kind and just in all His ways. His holy name be praised for ever. His paternal love is my solace, my staff and my support, and on it I rest my hope for your eternal destiny."

A Jewish mother's prayer in remembrance of her baby

Babes in Arms

Carry-cots, push-chairs, buggies and prams – these are the trappings of the modern baby in transit. But they are all relatively recent inventions. Queen Victoria first introduced the perambulator into English society in the nineteenth century. Soon every self-respecting infant was propped up in his own miniature carriage, usually propelled by a nanny.

Today, most parents' idea of "walking" the baby involves some kind of pushing device. So how did we manage before the arrival of the four-wheel drive? The answer is simple, but it works. Throughout humanity's history, babies have been carried in the arms of their care-givers. Chinese babies are transported in flowered, red cloths, which are still shaped like the animal skins our early ancestors would have used. Welsh babies traditionally "cutched up" (cuddled in) to their mothers in a large, crocheted shawl. This period of constant physical contact, widely known as the "in-arms phase", is a common feature of societies that value tactile communication.

Balinese babies are constantly held for their first 105 days, as they are believed to need physical contact to feel reassured in their new environment. Similarly, on the Japanese island of Okinawa, babies experience uninterrupted body contact with their mother or nursemaid: infants, as "gifts of the gods", are nurtured with boundless affection and indulgence.

There is evidence that being carried is more than just emotionally beneficial. Studies have shown that Ganda babies in East Africa, who are carried on their mothers' backs all day, are able to stand and walk much earlier than their American contemporaries. Research on the children of Inuit tribes has also uncovered a correlation between carrying and a child's development. A Netsilik baby of the Canadian Arctic is strapped to her mother's back with a special sash, which supports the infant under her buttocks. The baby is kept warm in a special hood in her mother's *attiggi* (a fur parka made for two) and she has a clear forward view either side of her

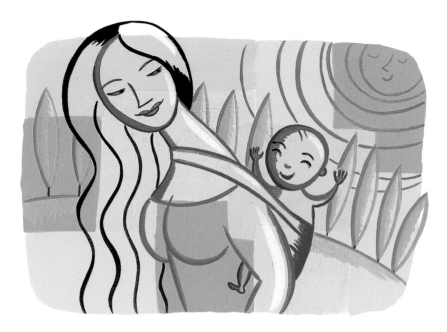

mother's head. Snug in her nest, the baby watches the world from a rapidly shifting vantage point as her mother moves around. Absorbing visual information from so many different and changing perspectives might explain the heightened spatial awareness of Inuit children. For example, they can often read a book upside-down as easily as the right way up.

Test results on the effects of holding babies have been so convincing that in Colombia modern doctors now promote skin-to-skin contact as a therapy for premature babies. Known as "kangaroo care", this technique is often used in preference to electronic incubation methods: the babies' health improves more quickly and parents can bond with their vulnerable babies.

Once you have her home, try carrying your baby in a sling for a day (specially designed slings are widely available to ensure safety) and experience the close-contact approach. She may seem heavy at first, but you will become accustomed to the weight. Your baby will gain confidence from your physical contact and will benefit from her new view of the world.

The Power of Touch

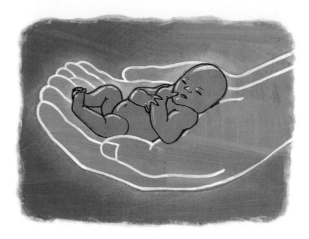

Born into a confusing world, with simple, primitive needs, all babies crave and respond to
human touch – scientists call this need "skin hunger". Babies are designed to be physically
appealing: a baby's soft skin compels us to stroke, kiss and protect him. When a baby gives vent
to an anguished wail he is often literally crying out to be held.

The Mundugumor of New Guinea raise their children with the minimum of contact. Infants are carried in baskets suspended from the mother's forehead, and at weaning they are pushed away from the breast and smacked. These actions may contribute to the aggressive behaviour valued by the tribe. But most cultures aim to encourage loving touch in their children. Babies' lives are shaped by the hands that hold them, and it is within our power to raise children who love to be held and to hold. The Filipino Tasay tribe live in a loving community, and the importance of touch is passed on through the generations. Babies are constantly stroked and held – even the adults sit arm in arm and nuzzle one another. The principles are so simple yet so effective: massage your baby, stroke his face as he feeds, and hold him in your arms as often as you can.

Baby Massage

Life in the womb is like a nine-month flotation, combined with an all-over body massage. Soothing massages can make a fractious newborn feel safe again. In India, where all children are massaged regularly, the art is passed down from mother to daughter; in Russian hospitals mothers are taught massage to stimulate the baby's immature nervous system. Moroccan babies are massaged with henna and butter, or an aromatic mixture including marjoram and mint. Nyinba babies in Nepal are massaged twice daily with mustard-seed oil and breastmilk.

Try giving your baby a gentle massage – a good time is after a warm bath and before sleep. First, spend time simply holding. When you are ready to begin, make sure that your hands are not cold: a Bornu baby in Nigeria is welcomed to the world with a massage from his birth attendants – but first they warm their hands over hot coals. Find a position that suits you both: your baby might lie against your chest, or with his back propped up on your raised thighs. Use cushions for support and soft music and lighting to create a relaxed atmosphere.

Smooth your baby's body with a light film of almond massage oil. (Essential oils are best avoided for baby massage.) Intuition is your best guide. Use your fingertips and keep all movements feather-light. Softly slide your hands in opposite directions across his stomach, and rotate your fingers clockwise around his belly button. Massage his legs, arms, fingers and toes. Avoid the cord stump in the early days, and do not pull on his limbs. Above all, watch and listen to your baby. If he becomes restless, he's had enough. Ten minutes of magical contact with his mother may be all he needs.

Tears and Smiles

*T*he crying comes first – a yell of anguish is usually the first signal of life. A baby's first breath takes five times more energy than all the other breaths to come. According to Native American Osage mothers, this cry is a prayer that the baby learned before her spirit descended to earth – she is calling to Grandfather Sun and Moon Woman to ask for their protection in her new world.

In many cultures a baby is encouraged to cry lustily to prove herself healthy. In Haiti, it was the custom for a large wooden bowl to be held upside-down over a sleepy newborn. This was beaten like a drum to make the baby wake up with a wail of distress. Until recently, Western doctors would hold babies up by their ankles and smack them to produce a loud cry and unblock the airways.

Other societies place emphasis on a gentle birth. French birth pioneer Frédéric Leboyer took many of his ideas from ancient India. Subtle lighting, whispering voices and the reassurance of the mother's body make it possible for some babies to be born without crying. The first breath is a sudden reflex, air rushes in and the baby exclaims. She is surprised, but not necessarily distressed.

A new baby does not weep real tears until around three weeks old, but her crying is a whole body experience – a rhythmical wail and a face completely distorted in the spasm of her own torment. All over the world, mothers soothe their crying babies by holding, suckling, rocking and singing to them. In Jamaica, as in many other cultures, older siblings are given the task of soothing the baby; girls stop their infant brother or sister from crying by strapping them to their backs and carrying them with them as they play.

In New Mexico, women of the Seri tribe have a solution for persistently crying babies. They take some twigs from the nest of a bird known as "the bird who sleeps in the afternoon". These are burned on four small fires placed at four corners around the restless child. As the smoke rises from

Among the Ibo peoples of western Africa, a newborn's cries are said to be plaintive songs to the unborn children whom he has left far behind in the spirit world.

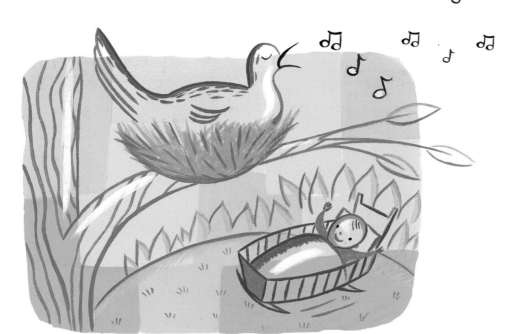

the flame, her mother sings an incan-
tation, calling on the bird's spirit to
ease her crying.

However much a baby cries, her
smiles are rarely very far behind. At
first, these magical, happy faces are
merely reflexes – fleeting expressions,
which may start as young as three
days old. According to an old Welsh
tradition, when a baby smiles or
laughs in her sleep, the fairies are
kissing her. Soon, however, your baby
offers her first real smile, a four-
week-old expression of delight. The
smiles become longer and broader,

until, at somewhere between four and
seven months old, she gives her first
specific, intentional and affectionate
smile. Now she is ready to laugh.

Laughter is perilously close to crying, a signal of relief, often resulting
from potentially scary games like
"peek-a-boo" or tickling. A laughing
baby sends the powerful message: "I
know I am safe with you." When she
realizes that she is in safe hands, her
cry becomes a chuckle. Soon, she
wants to repeat this pleasurable
experience, turning anticipated fear
into sheer joy.

Children of the Sky

*W*hen babies are born in twos, they bring twice the magic. Along the parched coastline of Delagoa Bay, in southeast Africa, twins of the Baronga tribe and their mothers are attributed with the power to bring rain. A mother of twins is known as *Tilo*, "The Sky", and her twins are known as "Children of the Sky". In spring, if the rains are late, Baronga women conduct a ritual to encourage the precious rain to fall. They put on grass skirts and sing wild songs; then they call at a house where twins have been born. Although fresh water is scarce, they drench the mother of twins with water carried in pitchers. Now that the Sky – a mother imbued with twin magic – is wet, the rains will come.

More twins are born to African mothers than to any other race in the world – one in every twenty-two African pregnancies is expected to result in twins, compared with one in a hundred for North Americans and Europeans, and one in two hundred for the Japanese.

Twin births are surrounded with mystery and super-stition. Some tribes assume that a woman must have had sex with two men at around the same time. Others see multiple births as an aberration, the work of evil spirits. And a few consider the intimacy of twins in the womb an impropriety which must be rectified – in Japan and the Philippines, boy–girl twins were tra-ditionally required to marry each other when they came of age.

Although twins were considered undesirable by some (the Navaho Native Americans likened twins to the litters of lower animals), elsewhere they were regarded as a great bless-ing. Kings of Benin would give any mother of twins the services of a royal wet nurse to indicate his plea-sure at their arrival. Ewe women of

West Africa wear a special badge to announce proudly that they have had twins. You could join them by making your own "Mother of Twins" badge (if you get a spare minute!).

In places where twins are believed to have magical powers, they are often accorded special treatment. Among the Ga people of Africa, great efforts are made to meet their every request to avoid causing them anger. Every year, a *ɣeleɣeli*, or thanksgiving yam-feast, is held in honour of the pampered pair. The next child to be born is named *Tawia* – the Ga believe that he or she has been "sent" by the gods in order to serve the twins; and *Tawia* must spend his or her life in devotion to their many and varied needs. Unsurprisingly, Ga parents regard twins as a mixed blessing.

On a practical level, twins need skilful management. Their births can be more complicated and their early lives can cause both physical and economic strain on family life. But as most "sky" mothers will testify, they also bring more than double the delight. Who knows? They may even bring the spring rain.

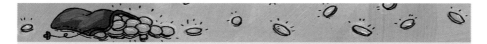

The Only Child

In many parts of the world, solitary children are rare. But in China, where government policy limits parents to one child, and in the West, where birth control is widely used, many families have only children. In America and Europe, for example, only children were five times more common in the 1990s than they were during the previous decade. Popular myth holds that a solitary child will be self-centred and inflexible, and is more likely to get divorced. But an intense upbringing with lots of praise (as well as lots of blame) need not cause problems – only children are usually conscientious and loyal. In European fairy tales, only children leave home to seek their fortune, returning with untold wealth. The moral may be that parents should take care to give their only child freedom to flourish fully.

Father Figures

The early stages of motherhood can seem like an inner sanctum, a private session for two. A new mother may be so absorbed with her baby that there is no obvious role for the new father. Many modern fathers struggle to define their role – they want to belong and to be useful, yet many feel excluded, both physically and emotionally, at this special time.

In many cultures, fatherhood confers a new status for a man, and significant post-natal roles are found for him. Kayapó men of Brazil are given a sudden elevation in social rank upon the birth of their first baby. Kayapó marriage is only considered to be fully consummated once a child is born; the "bachelor" officially becomes a husband and father and moves into his wife's household.

Other societies offer new fathers a rite of passage. In Japan, Ainu men go on a twelve-day retreat in order to meditate on their honourable state and new responsibility. In New Guinea, the young Arapesh men are initiated into fatherhood by an experienced father. The older man gives the new father a special herbal bath and paints him with white pigment. Then the initiate must catch himself an eel (a phallic emblem) to symbolize his entrance into the community of fathers.

There are many ways in which connections are made between a father and his baby. Often, the father's role takes on a protective quality. In the Congo, Mbuti fathers sprinkle their babies and wives with sacred vine juices to protect and strengthen them. Fathers in some societies like to sleep with the baby on their chests, which helps with bonding and fosters a sense of guardianship. It is the duty of the Muslim father to offer protection and hope to the newborn. He engages in a simple ritual with his baby by placing a piece of date in the child's mouth to show him how sweet life can be.

As a child grows up, fathers often begin to figure more prominently, supplementing and complementing the mother's role, as teacher and

To Day's End

With the night
the house grows dark,
with the night
comes candle light,
with the night
comes the end of play,
and with the night
comes Daddy home.

Traditional Welsh saying

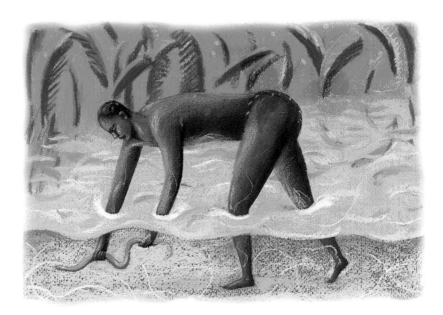

guide. Traditionally, mothering focuses on a child's inner needs, while fathering is expected to be more concerned with preparation for the world outside. For example, fathers have been shown to use a wider vocabulary when talking to a small child than mothers, who tend to use simpler, special language forms, such as "motherese" (see p.106). Studies have also shown that, although fathers (as a general rule) tend to spend less time with their children, they play with them more intensively and dramatically during the time that they have.

However, the behaviour of fathers, as that of mothers, tends to be culturally determined and is open to infinite possibilities. On the Maltese islands, where parental roles are strictly defined, a father's involvement in childcare may simply be to issue commands. By contrast, Balinese fathers are very gentle and spend more time than mothers looking after babies: even after feeding, which in many cultures is an important bonding time for mother and baby, Balinese babies are handed straight back to their fathers.

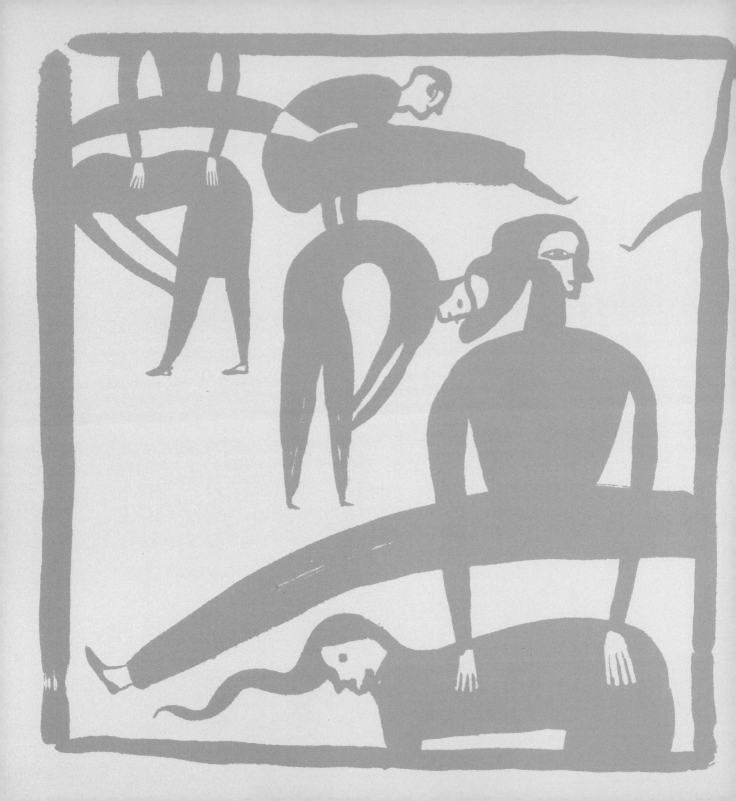

The Child Grows

The intense togetherness of the early months must fade,
but the passage through childhood brings with it new joys
and challenges. As the child grows, a unique character begins
to emerge with her own preferences and perspective on the
world. From infancy to adulthood, a child needs her parents
to balance their protective instincts with the need to let
go until, finally, she is grown.

First Foods

A baby's first taste of "real" food traditionally comes from his mother's milk, which absorbs and dilutes the flavours of the food that she eats. So breastfed babies start attuning to their future diet from the minute they take their first feed. Thai babies enjoy breastmilk infused with traces of lemon grass and galangal root, and older Indian babies may even be perfectly content to eat spicy curry. Recent research indicates that bottle-fed babies (who will not have had the benefit of food-traces in their mother's own milk) are less willing to accept solid food.

In some cultures, babies are given their first solid food soon after birth. Among the Karen tribe of northern Thailand, babies are fed a few grains of rice and told: "This is what you will be eating in a year's time." Babies in northern Canada and Greenland were traditionally given some meat at birth to initiate them into the cycle of exchange between humans and nature – it was believed that animals willingly gave up their lives in exchange for correct ritual obser-vance. Whether or not the baby ate the food was unimportant. The infant was not considered to be fully human until he had joined (ritually at least) the meat-sharing community.

Methods of weaning range from sweet temptations to abrupt deter-rents. Tchambuli infants in New Guinea are lured from the breast with sugar cane and lotus stems; but in Mexico, Aztec mothers called a sud-den halt to breastfeeding by smearing their nipples with crushed chillies.

Many babies have a combined diet of breastmilk and solid food until the age of two or three. According to numerous cultural and medicinal tra-ditions, the shift to solid foods is best made slowly to avoid losing the physical and emotional benefits of breastfeeding. In some tribal societies babies are breastfed for up to five or six years – the length of time breast-milk is designed to be fed to an in-fant. However, in some cultures

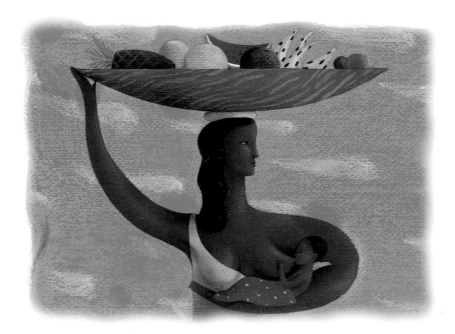

weaning takes place after a few months. In Western society this might be because the mother needs to return to work. Elsewhere, sudden weaning is believed to encourage certain characteristics in the child. Native American Plains tribes used a method of abrupt breast denial in the belief that doing so encouraged an aggressive temperament in their children, which in later life made them fierce and formidable warriors.

Many of us take for granted the ease and accessibility of a liquidizer with which we can pulp numerous varieties of readily available foods. First foods vary greatly from culture to culture, and they generally consist of whatever items are fresh, local and easily digested: African babies might begin with mashed banana; while babies from Mediterranean regions with mashed avocado. In many indigenous tribes, instead of mashing with kitchen equipment, mothers employ the traditional "kiss–feeding" method. The food is chewed into a pulp in the mother's own mouth before she transfers it to her baby's mouth with a kiss.

The Gift of Language

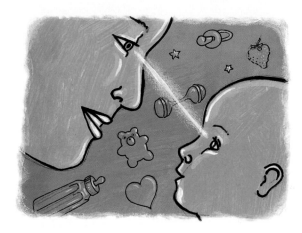

The Latin word infans, *from which we derive "infant", means "he who is unable to speak". But all mothers know that communication begins long before actual speech. Babies "talk" to us with their eyes, their expressions and their whole bodies, and we respond to them in the same language.*

The human race is set apart from other animals through our highly developed use of language and understanding. A baby can hear conversations even while she is in the womb. From the minute she is born she begins to filter the rhythms of her native tongue and gradually learns to recognize meaning. In South Africa, the Bantu tribe celebrate the first time a child answers to her name with a feast.

The best way to encourage your baby's language is to strike up a two-way conversation. Mothers all over the world talk to their babies in a special language, known as "motherese" or "baby talk". Without learning how, we tend use the simplest words, altering our grammar to make sentences shorter. Mothers talk of themselves in the third person, speak more slowly, repeat things, and speak to their infants in a sing-song pitch (children learn more easily through rhythm and song). By looking at our babies while we are talking to them, we also teach them the facial expressions that accompany speech.

Mama Papa

Babies start to babble from around three months, repeating easy syllables like "da", "ta", "ma", "ba" and "pa". All around the world these first basic sounds form the roots of common names for other family members, most importantly "mother" and "father". For example, *baba* means "mother" among the Gusii tribe of Kenya, while *baban* is "father" for the Sambarivo people of Madagascar. The English word "daddy" is *tata* in Greek, *tatas* in Sanskrit and *papa* in French.

Considering the amount of time she spends with her newborn in the first months, a mother might expect her baby to say her name first. But this rarely happens. Studies have shown that, from Africa to Slovenia, babies try to name their fathers before their mothers. Perhaps father, a familiar but often slightly more distant figure, is considered more worthy of mention (mother is just the fixture who meets the baby's every need – indeed she is perceived almost as an extension of the baby's own body). Or perhaps mothers deliberately choose to interpret their baby's first word as "daddy", in order to make a father feel more important and to add further proof of his paternity.

In Europe, the origins of the colloquial words for mother are intimately connected with breastfeeding. Mom, Mam, Mummy, Maman, Mutti, Mama – all these words derive from the ancient Greek *mamman*, which means "to cry for the breast", and the Roman *mamma*, meaning "breast". (In English, the glands in the breasts are called "mammaries".)

Before you know it, your baby will be giving her own special names to her brothers and sisters and the cat. But it's hardly surprising that a baby's very first syllables are directed at her parents – the first objects of a baby's attention.

Following a Fashion

African children in very remote tribes are usually given the freedom to roam shoeless and without a stitch of clothing. Unhampered by physical restrictions, or the need to keep clothes clean, they move confidently and easily in their own skin. Having begun life without even a diaper or nappy, young children are allowed to wander in all their natural beauty for their first few years.

This is in stark contrast with the trussed-up offspring of European gentry of the past. A seventeenth-century swaddled baby wore a linen shirt; a long bellyband for stomach support; a fine diaper or nappy square; a large rectangular wrap or "bed" to hold his arms against his sides; swaddling bands; another "bed"; and finally a "stayband" to keep his head straight. This textile parcel was topped off with two linen caps and a triangular decoration known as a "biggin". The result was a generation of babies who were passive and immobilized.

Children's clothes were often used as status symbols for wealthy families. In Victorian England, it was fashionable to dress little boys as sailors and cavaliers, or as miniature Scotsmen, complete with kilt and sporran. Girls were robed in many layers of petticoats and crinolines just like their mothers.

People often went to great lengths to make their babies look older so that they might escape bewitchment by fairies. European Christening gowns are traditionally twice as long as the baby, so that evil spirits will be fooled into thinking that an older, less vulnerable child is on his way to church. Anbarra Aborigines smear their newborn babies with ashes and charcoal for a similar reason. Their infants are light skinned and become darker as they grow – the black camouflage averts evil spirits said to be attracted to young babies.

In many cultures, children are painted with bright colours. Nuba women of Sudan paint the crowns of

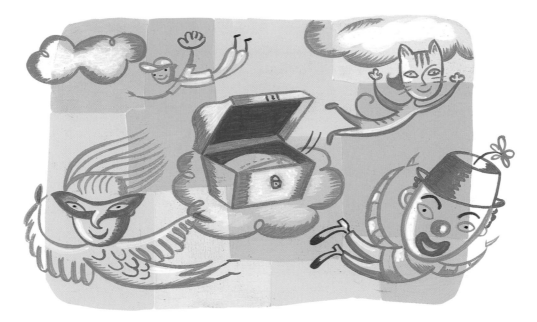

their babies' heads with oil and red or yellow ochre, the pattern proclaiming the family group to which the child belongs. Older children are adorned with intricate facial markings denoting their age and kin groups. Australian Aboriginal children are decorated with ancient markings (with secret meanings) for the enactment of Dreamtime stories relating events at the beginning of the world.

From around the ages of three or four, when their imaginations have really started to develop, most children love to have their faces painted. Try it, and see how absorbed your child becomes as you paint on a whole new personality. This form of "dressing up" allows a transformation more complete than merely putting on new clothes. For a few hours, your child can enter a fantasy world of his own, in which he actually becomes a tiger or a clown.

Keep a well-stocked dressing-up box, full of old clothes and shoes (remove loose buttons or high heels if necessary), hats made of cardboard, and old bits of jewellery or old watches. This is a wonderful land of make-believe in a box, which will stimulate your child's imagination.

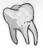
Tooth Tales

*T*eeth are landmarks on the path from infancy to adulthood, but their schedules of arrival and departure vary from child to child. One in 2,000 babies is born with a tooth, yet there are one-year-olds who seem to manage with empty gums. Count your child's teeth on her first birthday – an old English tradition holds that the number reveals how many brothers and sisters she will have.

A child's first tooth is a milestone that mothers everywhere anticipate with great eagerness. In Uganda, the Dhagga tribe holds a special ritual for its arrival. "Now," they say, "the child is complete." Grandma rubs herbs into the baby's gums, blesses her to encourage a healthy set of teeth and gives her a first taste of solid food.

First teeth (usually the four front teeth) cause few problems for babies, but the arrival of molars may make them miserable. To ease teething pains, rub maple syrup mixed with a few drops of chamomile oil into your baby's gums. You could also try massaging the web between the thumb and index finger (the acupressure point for toothache). It is a myth that teething causes fever and rashes, but keep a look out for one bright red cheek and excessive dribbling.

Children's teeth usually appear two by two, upper incisors followed by the lower pair. At the age of six or seven, children lose their "milk" (or "baby") teeth to make room for their adult set. Chinese children bury their upper baby teeth in the ground, to encourage their upper adult teeth to grow downward, while they throw their lower baby teeth over the roof of the house, so that their bottom adult teeth will shoot upward.

Many children are recompensed for the loss of baby teeth. In Britain, each fallen tooth is placed under the

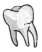

child's pillow or on a plate with some salt. As the child sleeps, the "tooth fairy" exchanges the tooth for a coin. It is sometimes said that the transfer must take place before midnight or bad luck will follow. In Italian tradition, children leave their baby teeth in the fireplace. During the night a "mouse" takes the tooth away and leaves a sweet, or a coin, in its place. In homes without a fireplace, teeth are left on the window sill, and these days a coin, rather than a sweet, is the more common reward. In Spain, gifts are left under the child's pillow by Ratoncito Perez, "Perez, the little

mouse", in exchange for baby teeth. Balinese parents hold joyful ceremonies to mark the loss of baby teeth. When adult teeth arrive, the child is said to have completed the long transition from the spirit to the human world. Some people say that the change of teeth is a mini-adolescence for a child. Watch out for mood swings and sensitivity.

The setting of teeth in a child's mouth also has its own lore. In Scottish tradition, a gap between the two front teeth is lucky; but if all the teeth are set too widely apart, in the future the child will have to leave her home town to seek her fortune.

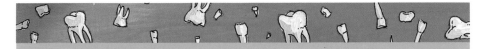

Protecting the Ivory Towers

Brushing teeth morning and night with toothpaste is a ritual most common in Western societies, which have a love affair with refined sugar. Norwegian children are taught to fear TanVerk Trollet, the toothache troll, who will move into their mouths if they neglect to brush their teeth. But in Zaire, sweets, and so tooth decay, are extremely rare. Children clean their teeth

with chew sticks, which they break off from the Peelu or "toothbrush" tree.

Until your child is six or seven, she will probably need help with cleaning her teeth. You could encourage regular brushing by joining in at the same time. Most children love to take part in activities with their parents (at this early age) – and your own teeth will benefit, too!

Once Upon a Time

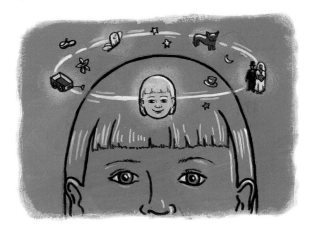

Many Westernized parents have lost faith in their ability to tell a story without a script. Yet children are appreciative listeners and enjoy the simplest of attempts. To rediscover the ancient skills of oral history, try retelling simple family events. They might be funny or dramatic, featuring, say, grandpa when he was a young boy, or the funniest moments from a family wedding.

A child's inner world needs regular exercise. Television and picture books do too much of the work, stunting the powers of the imagination. Tell a child a story, and he will create his own screen of pictures, as vivid for him as every-day life. To an open-hearted child, fables and fairy stories carry the weight of emotional truth and transport him into realms of limitless possibility, where good and evil, bravery and cowardice, ambition and humility do battle.

Stories teach, entertain and forge a unique bond between the teller and the child. In many societies, young people learn their cultural heritage at their grandmothers' knee. The Swedish poet Selma Lagerlf said that her grandmother sat all day long in a corner, waiting to tell children fairy stories. The old lady would end the stories by placing her hand on the young child's head and saying: "All this is true, as I can see you and you are seeing me."

The Art of Storytelling

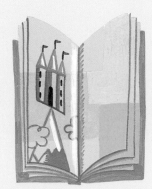

Between the ages of two and three, children love to hear stories about things that they know: retellings of their daily routines and familiar people help them to build up trust in what they see. You can tell your child stories about almost anything in his world: the ducks in the park, the cat next door. Children also respond to the repetition and rhythm of nursery rhymes, and will love to hear stories of your childhood.

Around the age of four, children are ready to enter fully into worlds of make-believe. You could begin by reading stories from books, but all children love to be told special stories invented just for them. Anthologies of traditional folk and fairy tales, such as those by the German Brothers Grimm, or the *Arabian Nights*, offer a valuable source of inspiration.

Memorizing a tale, as all traditional storytellers do, is not as difficult as you might think. Read the story several times out loud and visualize the action. Practise retelling each part. Adapt the storyline of any fairy tale for your own child by introducing familiar figures or places from his life, taking care not to make the story too frightening – in fairy tales dangers and quandaries are always resolved happily.

Modify your voice to bring your story alive: whisper secrets that the "bad guys" must not hear; use croaky or booming sounds for dangerous characters; brave and bold language for heroes and heroines. Change pace with the unfolding action: slow and with suspense when danger lurks near; steady and sure when resolution seems imminent. Make eye contact with your child and use facial expressions for emphasis. You are literally an actor playing all the parts and your child is the fully absorbed and captivated audience.

Marking Time

In the West, traditional birthday celebrations have been handed down from the birthday rituals of the ancient Greeks. The birthday cake, nowadays ever more elaborate, in its original form was simply round and white to honour the full moon – a symbol of regeneration and growth.

Evil spirits were traditionally thought to linger at birthday celebrations, and rituals to ward them off still survive. In England, the birthday child is given "the bumps" (his friends grasp the child's arms and legs and lift her high into the air for each year of her life, ending with a gentle bump on the ground); in Scotland she is given a soft birthday punch; and in Belgium, to wake her up, she is given a gentle needle prick.

However, not all cultures regard calendar time as the most significant marker of a child's growth. Hupa and Omaha Native American tribes believed that counting was wicked, and so had little idea of dates and the linear passage of years as we know them. Australian Anbarra Aborigines describe childhood as passing through certain stages of behaviour: *Wupa* (the "baby inside") grows into *Yokoko* (the "tiny one"). At three to six weeks, the baby is known as "the smile". Later she becomes "she who sits on the shoulder"; the "frightened one"; and (at around three years old) the "cheeky one". From about five years the child joins the "kid's gang" until pre-puberty when boys are called "the big ones" and girls are known as "the breasts". In Samoa, celebratory feasts are held when babies learn how to sit, crawl and stand. Elsewhere, rituals such as head-shaving, ear-piercing and circumcision mark the transition from childhood to adulthood.

Nevertheless, celebrating the anniversary of a child's birth is the most widely practised method of marking growth. The song "Happy Birthday" originated in the USA, but is now sung all over the world in different languages. Many cultures have their own original songs too: in Venezuela *Hoy es Tu Día* ("Today is Your Day") and in Holland *Lang Zal Hij Leven* ("Long May He Live") ring out in celebration for the birthday boy or girl.

If you have a birthday party for your child, you could adapt the following game from Central America. In the original game, the birthday child has to break the *piñata*, a decorated bag of treats which is attached to a rope, suspended from a beam or hook in the ceiling. The child is blindfolded and twirled around to disorient her. An adult places the rope over the beam to hold the bag aloft, raising and lowering it while the child tries to hit the *piñata* with a stick. Ask your party guests to stand in a line while you suspend the *piñata* appropriately and securely. Let each guest take a turn at hitting the *piñata* and whoever breaks the bag can win a special prize. If you fill the bag with sweets, then everyone can share the *piñata*'s gifts.

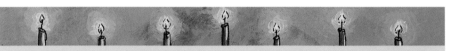

The Candle of Life

When you light your child's birthday candles, you are actually celebrating her safe journey through another year. The ritual dates back to medieval Germany, when birthday candles were kept alight all day. Eventually, German families introduced small candles to put on top of the birthday cake – one for each year, plus one for the day of birth. This extra birthday flame is the Candle of Life. If a child could blow all her candles out at once, symbolically wiping out the past and starting afresh, her wish would be granted (as long as it was kept secret). The candle smoke was believed to carry her secret desire to the heavens.

Some German children are given a twelve-year-candle as a christening present. You could decorate a large candle for your own child, using a pen and stickers to mark twelve stages. On each birthday, let the candle burn down to the next line to show the relevant year.

Skills for Life

Young supple limbs and willing hearts play an important role in the running of many societies. Throughout history, adults have found work to occupy their offspring, and each community is careful to hand on its required life skills to growing children. In Bolivia, young people are expected to help with the cultivation of the most important crop – potatoes. In Alaska, boys learn to hunt moose and caribou with their fathers from an early age. From the hill-tribe villages of Vietnam to the islands of Indonesia, children collect firewood, chop it and carry it home. In many places, agile children climb coconut trees to harvest the nuts. Many parents rely on their children to help with these time-consuming, essential tasks.

In Tudor Britain, children of rich families were "placed out" with families of similar rank to learn manners and household duties. The system was a kind of apprenticeship that began when a child reached the age of seven or eight and lasted for seven years. Children would be required to perform menial but supposedly "character-building" tasks, with the aim of ensuring that, by the time a child reached adolescence, he had learned to behave appropriately and appreciatively under any circumstances.

Sharing responsibility for the running of a household, growing and preparing food, and caring for younger children are the kinds of tasks that help to teach older children discipline and give them a sense of belonging. However, for most children in developed nations, "learning" takes place in a school building. Of course, school educates children in social understanding and interaction, but often the routine of processing information all day and having to do private study in the evenings, means that fewer children nowadays benefit from both school and home "work". In rural Lebanon a wonderful compromise is reached which gives children a

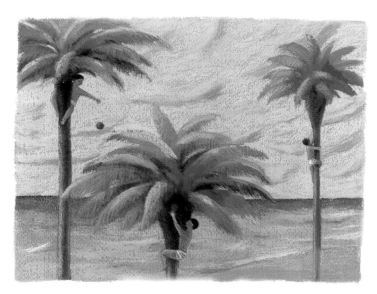

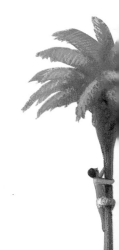

full range of life skills. Children gather at the "school under the oak tree" with the village priest to learn writing, mathematics, geography and so on, as well as to learn how to interact with their peers; but they go back home during the middle of the day to eat with their families and help out with daily chores, such as fetching water, cooking and weaving.

You may well not need or wish your child to "work", but all children love feeling important and that their role in the family is significant. By finding and creating easy, but worthwhile tasks for your child, you will encourage him to feel a valued and useful member of the family. Helpful chores could include: pairing socks after they have been washed; shelling peas into a bowl; giving a cake mix a "special stir" with a wish to make it rise; collecting the mail in the mornings; pulling weeds from the garden; putting crumbs out for the birds during the winter. All these small "jobs" will encourage your child to feel capable and special. They may even make him inclined to think of his own ways of being helpful.

Whatever the nature of a child's work, when it is finished, all children spend their free time engaged in the much more serious business of play.

Games Children Play

In the Philippines, it is said that when a boy is born, the trees and the birds are sad, because he will climb the trees, pick their fruits and catapult the birds. When a girl is born, the flowers are sad, because she will pick them.

Play is a universal feature of childhood. In many ways, it is the "work" of growing up. Through jumping and chasing, guessing and imagining, children develop invaluable skills that will help them make their journey into adult life. For example, the popular game of Hide-and-Seek (or Hide-and-Go-Seek) exercises a child's physical and mental faculties, calling upon memory skills, spatial awareness, problem solving and, most important of all, social interaction.

Games and songs are handed down through the generations with amazingly few changes. Maori children still act out (as a chasing game) the myth of the moon and the goddess Rona: the two fought causing the moon's waxing and waning. As if to prove that there really is an international human language, the pastimes of one culture are often to be found duplicated thousands of miles across the globe in another. Take, for example, the game of Tag, otherwise known as "Tig" or "It", among hundreds of other names. In sunny countries, such as Saudi Arabia, children dodge each others' shadows. Shadows play a part in Spain too, where children play a form of Tag known as "Moon and Morning Stars". One child, the Moon, must stay inside the shadow of a large tree. Other children are Morning Stars who taunt the Moon until they are "tagged".

The simple act of jumping has also become the basis for hundreds of different games found all over the world. Children everywhere enjoy skipping, or "jumping rope", with

The bright moon and the morning stars,
The bright moon and the morning stars,
Where the light shines gay
We dance and play,
But who will venture into the shadow?

A chant for the Spanish children's game "Moon and Morning Stars" their friends. A Chinese game *Tiao pi jin* ("elastic rope") involves two children standing opposite each other anchoring a single, taut loop of elastic around their ankles. A third child jumps into and out of the loop, and if he reaches the other side without touching the elastic, the loop is brought further up the legs of the two anchors, forcing the subsequent jump to be higher. The loop is pulled up a little higher each time, until the jumping child touches the elastic. The "jumper" than becomes an anchor and one of the anchors takes a turn to jump (and so on until all three children have had a turn at jumping). The winner is the person who jumped the highest. A comparable game in Africa sees children jumping over increasing distances, marked out by sticks.

Many other children's games have a surprising antiquity. Ancient Greek vases show children playing with yo-yos; kites were flown in Japan thousands of years ago, yet are still a common sight on a breezy day. In ancient Rome, children played with toy houses, hoops and spinning tops, and romped on see-saws and swings.

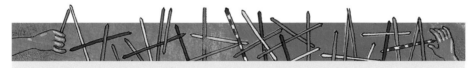

Pick-up Sticks

Whether we call it "Pick-up Sticks", "Spillikins" or "Jackstraws", this game of skill was originally played with bamboo sticks in ancient China, where it was called *liu bo*. You need forty dowels the diameter of a toothpick (available from hardware stores), cut into 9in (23cm) lengths. Sharpen the ends with a pencil sharpener. Then, paint twenty sticks yellow; ten, red; five, blue; three, green; and two with stripes.

To play, bunch the sticks in one hand, set them upright on a smooth surface and release them suddenly. Each player must pick up one stick at a time from the pile. If any other stick is disturbed, it is the next player's turn. Striped sticks, once retrieved, can be used to tease out other sticks. Give three points for each yellow stick; five points for red; ten points for blue; fifteen for green, and twenty for the stripes.

Goodness and Mischief

Some societies don't have a concept of naughtiness. It is believed that if children have inner discipline, stemming from a deep sense of responsibility and group connection, they will rarely need punishment. Ainu children in Japan are regarded as "children of the gods" and, as such, are treated with great affection and indulgence until the age of seven. Literally, they can do no wrong.

Many Western notions of behaviour stem from a Christian belief that children are "sinners" at heart and that external discipline must be imposed. In Victorian England it was believed that – in a world of complex social etiquette – children were not capable of behaving well without physical persuasion. "Spare the rod," they said, "and spoil the child."

Many parents in other parts of the world would shudder to see the daily battle between parents and children in the West. Tribal life, which requires co-operation for survival, would be intolerable if parents were reduced to hitting, screaming and constant nagging. Most village cultures find other, more amenable, ways to transmit the rules.

Firstly, the rules of society are often handed down humourously, a part of the evening's entertainment. Oral history offers morals and life lessons for children to heed. Australian Aboriginal children learn this way when they sit around the fireside and hear stories of their ancestors during the Dreamtime.

Secondly, an established system of behaviour means that everyone knows what is expected, and dissent from the norm is rare. Among the Ngoni of East Africa, youngsters are taught impeccable manners from the age of five. They must sit correctly and always walk in front of their elders as it is considered rude to walk behind.

As she walks ahead, a child bends slightly forward with the words "I am before your eyes." Around the house, Ngoni girls help with chores, while boys sit with elders during council meetings and court proceedings.

Thirdly, children are expected to work their way into the community and learn by copying their elders. In most tribes, older children are expected to care for their younger siblings, help with family meals and tend livestock and crops.

Finally, children are given a potent mixture of freedom and responsibility.

After they have finished their chores children are free to roam with their peers, learning self-direction and enjoying adult-free adventures.

Discipline is a crucial part of a child's education. However, it is easy to imagine that this means imposing set rules and punishments, when in fact children learn more readily by example and through encouragement. Learn to notice your child's co-operative behaviour, describe and praise her best efforts, and she will reward you with her own instinctive desire to please.

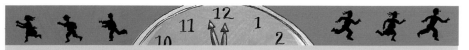

The Noon-day Witch

A cautionary tale from Prague

There once was a mother and father and a boy, who lived together in a single room. The Mother worked hard and often became very tired. One day, when her son was misbehaving, she lost her patience and threatened him. "If you are not good," said the Mother, "the Noon-day Witch will come and carry you away." She didn't really mean it, but she hadn't noticed the Noon-day Witch watching through the long, thin gap in the door.

The boy carried on moping and whining, and so, on the strike of twelve, the Noon-day Witch sneaked into the house to take him away. Suddenly, the father arrived home from fetching water and scared off the Witch just in time. She escaped through the window, knocking over a flower pot in her haste. Even today in the Czech republic, some people still don't let children go out at noon, for fear of the Noon-day Witch.

Trial By Fever

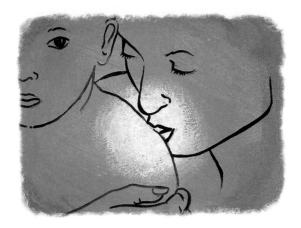

A touch of magic has always helped to make children feel better. When children fall and bump themselves, they often run to their parents for a kiss. "Kissing to make better" derives from the ancient ritual of sucking out the evil that was believed to cause pain.

Without the benefit of medical centres or doctors, women from remote tribes become highly adept at assessing illness. A survey of native Mexican mothers showed that they could diagnose a wide range of conditions just from looking at a child's eyes (as in Western iridology). They also believe, like Western homoeopaths, that a child emerges strengthened from his "trial by fever".

Mothers all over the world treat common children's illnesses with traditional remedies made from herbs and plants that grow nearby. You, too, can ease many childhood ailments with herbal remedies – for example, hyssop for asthma, elderflower and licorice for coughs and catarrh or Californian Poppy for sleeplessness. Chamomile, peppermint and cinnamon can be used for digestive upsets, and yarrow and catmint to regulate a fever. Consult a reputable herbal practitioner to help you get started in the art of natural healing.

Treating Like with Like

Homoeopathy, a system of "subtle energy" healing, takes its name from two Greek words: *homos* (meaning "same as") and *pathos* (meaning "suffering"). In other words, homoeopathy works on the principle of "treating like with like", to try to trigger the body into self-healing.

In homoeopathic remedies, the curative substance is "sub-molecular" – it is diluted until there is no actual substance left. All that remains is the "water-memory" of the original substance, which, even for plants or minerals that might otherwise be toxic, is completely harmless in this form.

Today, homoeopathy is a popular choice of treatment for parents who do not want their children to take strong medicines. For example, if a child has a fever (hot, flushed skin and glassy eyes), he may be given the water-memory dose of Belladonna, a substance that would cause fever if given in large quantities to a healthy person. For absolute safety it is best to consult a reputable homoeopathic practitioner before giving any remedies (which should be individually designed for each patient) to your child.

Some of the most common homoeopathic curatives for common childhood ailments include Aconite, Arnica, Chamomilla and Pulsatilla (all of these can be found in the form of a powder or granules). Aconite is used to reduce the effects of the sudden onset of illness, and anxiety, fever, coughs and croup. Arnica is wonderful for healing bruises (including "emotional bruising"). Pulsatilla can soothe children who are feeling weepy. Chamomilla is the first choice for earache or teething pain and can also be given to a restless child who has difficulty sleeping.

Rites of Passage

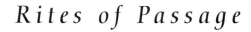

*I*n almost every culture, there is formal provision to mark a child's "coming of age" – a ceremony that celebrates achievement and bids farewell to childhood. Rites of passage give children a psychological stepping stone from the familiar world of childhood to the new challenges of adult life.

In Western society, a ceremonial key to the front door, depicted on typical twenty-first-birthday cards, is the symbol for the end of childhood and full entry into the world outside the home. Many young people in the West find that becoming an adult is not a triumphant arrival, but rather a drawn-out process characterized by confusion and self-doubt. Perhaps holding a ceremony at the beginning of adolescence, around the age of thirteen, rather than at its symbolic "end" at twenty-one (or eighteen as it is in many countries) helps children to acknowledge that puberty is just the beginning of the long journey to becoming a "grown up".

Some children are expected to endure physical pain to demonstrate their readiness to assume the status of adulthood. In South America, the remote Yequana tribe ask all their young people (girls as well as boys) to take one or two lashes of the whip in public at puberty.

In other cultures, adolescent rites of passage take the form of a spiritual awakening. The Native American tribes of the Plateau region encouraged children to gain spiritual power from visions and dreams. Upon puberty, boys and girls would retreat to a remote place in order to seek a vision. These vigils could last years before the spirits revealed themselves. The young person would often keep the spiritual knowledge that they had gained secret throughout their lives.

In Jewish tradition, a boy's Bar Mitzvah (which takes place on his thirteenth birthday) is a momentous event. After years of study, a boy assumes his obligation of observing Jewish law. During the Bar Mitzvah

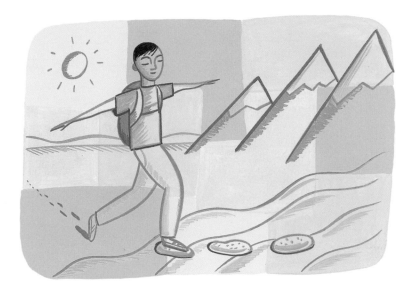

ceremony in the synagogue, he is expected to chant, for the first time, a section from the text of ancient Hebraic law, the *Torah*.

Balinese girls, rather than boys, are the centre of attention during puberty rituals. The Balinese place great value on childbearing, and the first sign of menstruation is a time of celebration. Girls are ritually wedded to Sanghyang Semara-Ratih, the god of beauty and sexual congress, who has the power to cure disease and bring good luck. During the ceremony, they must demonstrate their homely skills of spice-grinding and rice-pounding.

If you would like to acknowledge and celebrate your child's approaching adulthood with a special "rite of passage", you could build in elements of preparation, reassurance and self-discovery. We cannot, as many tribal peoples can, provide a single vision of what growing up entails. Our society has many routes, and it is ultimately up to our children to choose their own. We nurture, we educate, we control for a while – but in the end, we hand over power. If we have prepared our children well enough, and sent them off with our blessing, then they will have the strength to find their own place in the world.

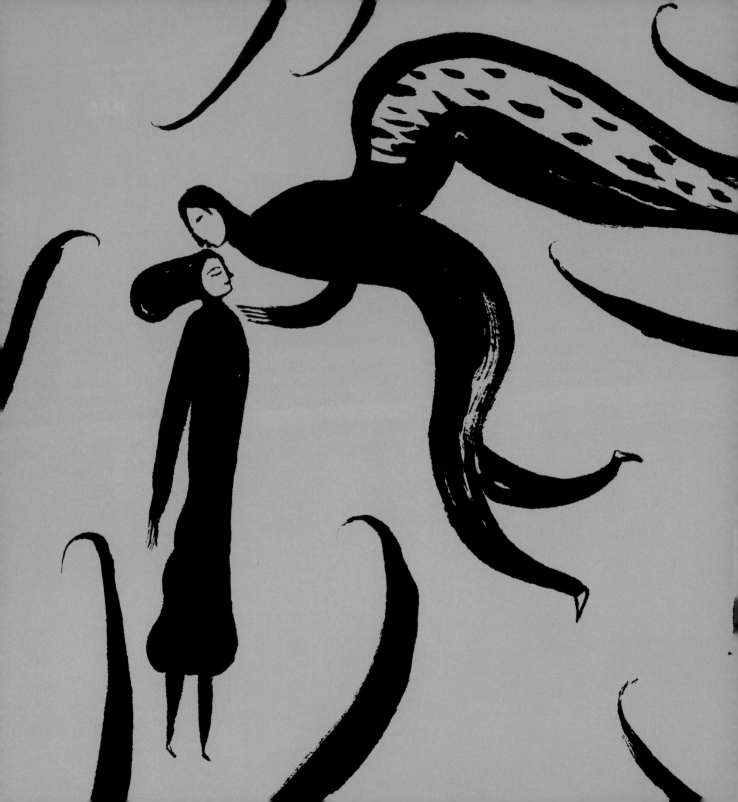

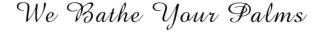

We Bathe Your Palms

We bathe your palms
in showers of wine,
in the crook of the kindling,
in the seven elements,
in the sap of the tree,
in the milk of the honey.

We place nine, pure choice gifts
in your clear beloved face:
the gift of form,
the gift of voice,
the gift of fortune,
the gift of goodness,
the gift of eminence,
the gift of charity,
the gift of integrity,
the gift of true nobility,
the gift of apt speech.

A traditional Gaelic blessing for a young person leaving home

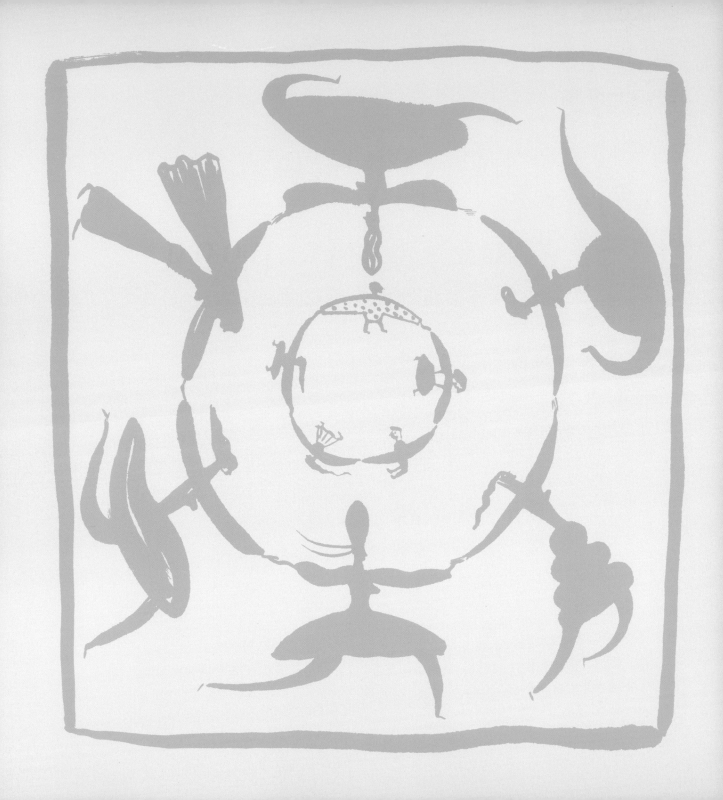

The Sisterhood of Mothers

Mothers are the guardians of life – they embody the mysterious regeneration that sustains all humanity. Their wealth of inherited wisdom is transmitted down through the generations, from mother to daughter, all over the world. Motherhood is a common cause, a universal and cherished gift, and an experience to share.

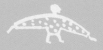

A Mother's Many Roles

Deep in the Amazon, where Kayapó Indians have lived relatively undisturbed for centuries, the roles of men and women are starkly divided. Men hunt and fish for food. And the women undertake almost everything else. They cultivate and harvest crops; gather, distribute and cook food; and hand-spin cotton. While they do all the household chores, they also look after the children, carrying their youngest infants on their backs.

In male-dominated tribal societies (such as many Australian Aboriginal groups), as well as in societies where women enjoy sexual equality (among the !Kung of Botswana, for example), women also often seem to do the bulk of the work. In most hunter-gatherer tribes, the women provide most of the food: they breastfeed the babies, gather edible roots and berries and catch small animals to sustain their families on a daily basis. The masculine activity of game-hunting is a risky and time-consuming process, requiring the manufacture of weapons and long expeditions. But it is not relied upon as a family's primary source of nourishment.

In societies such as these, mothering has to be regarded more as a sideline rather than an all-consuming task – survival depends upon the flexibility of the community, including mothers. Breastfeeding continues throughout other daily activities and babies are carried around all day in slings, freeing up their mothers' arms and hands for other tasks.

Women in tribal cultures develop many special skills in addition to household and mothering work. Native American women are highly skilled in a wide variety of crafts such as weaving, sewing, beadwork, midwifery, wood carving, and herbal

Wash on Monday

Iron on Tuesday

Mend on Wednesday

Churn on Thursday

Clean on Friday

Bake on Saturday

Rest on Sunday

A traditional English
mother's week

medicine. Few tribal women give up their other skills to devote themselves to motherhood – childcare is shared.

In Western society, too, the role of mother lies far beyond simply looking after the children. Even though the boundaries between a mother's and father's roles are now less defined, it still usually falls to the mother to undertake the essential household chores and be the primary caregiver. In addition, many women find themselves (through necessity or for self-fulfilment) having to take a regular job. As a result, many working mothers feel torn between their conflicting roles. Better nursery care and more flexible working environments are helping to bridge the gap between motherhood and career, but mothers everywhere still have to juggle their other commitments and tasks with childcare.

A mother's many roles can be all-consuming, so it is important that you take time to relax and congratulate yourself on a regular basis: to be a mother is to be a superwoman, and you deserve to be pampered every now and then.

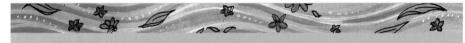

Your Own Time and Space

Some new mothers find it hard to take time for themselves without feeling guilty, but it is important not to let the many roles of motherhood overwhelm you physically and emotionally. Just a few minutes of calm can restore your sense of inner peace.

While your child is sleeping, take the opportunity to try a three-minute meditation. Count slowly from one to four, breathing in deeply as you do so.

Exhale in one long, slow out-breath. Do this five times, taking care not to over-breathe.

Immersing yourself in warm water is a wonderful way to escape. While your partner or a friend is on hand to childmind, take a luxurious bath. Sprinkle a few drops of lavender oil in the water. Rest your head on a towel, close your eyes, let your body dissolve into the water and unwind from the pressures of the day.

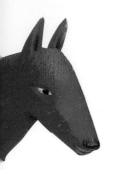

It Takes a Village

*T*here is a popular saying in the West: "It takes a village to raise a child." The task of bringing up children is diverse and, as much as it is joyful, it is also hard work – mothers need support. Today we tend to shy away from requesting help, especially when it comes to our children, fearing that it is a sign of our own failure. Nothing could be further from the truth. Throughout history, human beings have been interdependent, forming intimate networks of trust: asking for assistance when they need it and knowing that help, without judgment, is on hand.

Traditionally, in rural communities all over the world, the same childcare pattern is repeated: a mother provides the focus for her baby's needs, but an army of willing volunteers is available to give whatever support may be necessary. In places where a mother is given full respect for her essential work, the community gathers round to support her role. Among the Gusii tribe in Kenya, a woman's mother-in-law is in charge of her first birth, with wives of her husband's brothers and uncles all helping out. In addition, a large crowd of older women assemble at the door at the time of birth to welcome the new addition to the community and to give support and advice.

Generations of multi-tasking mothers have managed to combine childcare and other work without gadgets, supermarkets and automobiles. Instead, they rely on each other. Babies are raised not by one mother alone but by a team of mothers and helpers. Among the Tchambuli of New Guinea, for example, a child addresses all women in the tribe as *aiyai*, "mother". As far as he is concerned, their continued care means that they are worthy of the respect and affection he gives his real mother.

In many cultures even the task of breastfeeding is shared among friends, aunts and grandmothers. This ancient occupation of wet-nursing is often said to create a lasting connection between the nurse and the baby.

"Never doubt that a small group of thoughtful, committed citizens can change the world; indeed, it's the only thing that ever does."

Margaret Mead
(American anthropologist)

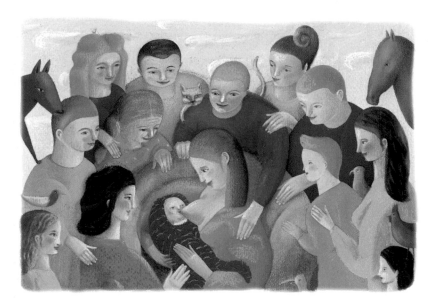

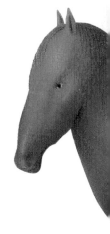

Among the Tausog peoples in the Philippines, children who are breast-fed by the same woman are *magsaw-duru*, "milk-brothers" (or milk-sisters) for ever. In other countries, a woman who breastfeeds her friend's baby becomes the child's mother-in-spirit.

Traditionally, carrying, bathing, feeding and cuddling are carried out by many members of the child's community, especially godparents, who develop a special relationship with the child. It is not always easy for us to create such a sense of community, especially now that we often find our own families geographically dispersed. So it is up to us to seek out a nearby network of support, and create our own "village" around us. Try enlisting the help of the teenager or the grandmother-figure next door, and other local mothers, who will offer support and understanding. Your "village" can be anyone who loves your child and is happy to give time. Apart from the benefits to your own well-being, a child who is surrounded by loving care-givers will feel secure, confident and able to interact easily with others – valuable characteristics that will equip him well for his future.

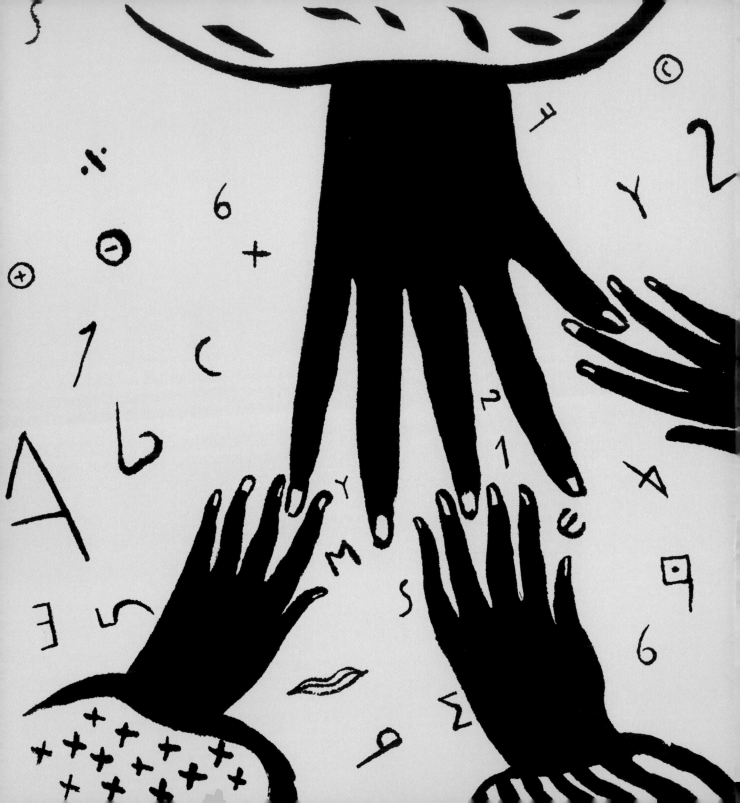

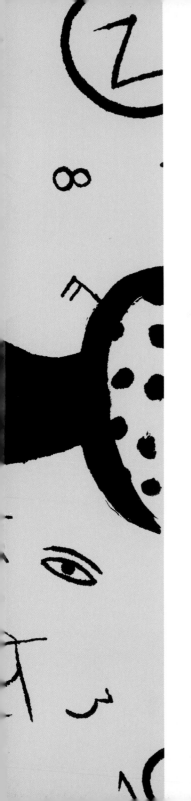

If You
Teach a Woman

"If you teach a man you teach one person;
if you teach a woman you teach a whole family."

Traditional saying from Kerala, southern India

The Mother-Line

The art and skills of motherhood are transmitted subtly through the generations. As one British grandmother highlights, "I only realized the power of the mother-line when I heard my daughter singing a lullaby to her baby – it was a lullaby taught to me by my own grandmother."

Girls all over the world spend much of their early childhood watching their mothers, absorbing their example and imitating their tasks. When new babies are born, older girls often carry them and care for them, earning the title "little mother".

Among the Zaramo of Tanzania, continuity between the generations of women is nurtured and guarded with pride. Girls stay close to the women in the household throughout their childhood and participate in all their work. They follow their mothers to fetch water from the well, balancing small tins on their heads until they are old enough to manage large water pots. Later on, they plant, tend and harvest crops, and look after their younger siblings. They learn to weave colourful hats and braid hair into intricate plaits; these crafts are shrouded in secrecy from men, and this fosters an atmosphere of mystery and pride in the whole sphere of "women's work".

Zaramo families consider the birth of a girl to be lucky, as one day she will bring bride-wealth to the family and ensure the continuation of the mother's line (which takes precedence over the father's). As a gesture of respect to the mother's parents, a firstborn girl is named after her maternal grandmother, and the girl is believed to share some of her grandmother's personal qualities.

In the Lebanon, when five generations of women from the same family gather together, it is called *Ya sette kellme settik* ("Oh grandmother speak to your grandmother"). The physical gathering of the mother-line – a daughter with her mother, grandmother, great-grandmother, and so on – represents a vast store of mothering wisdom and experience.

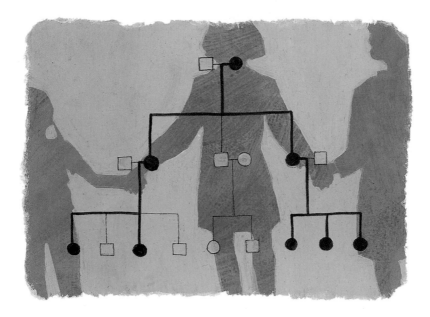

Of course, knowledge and experience are only passed on if the values of the past are respected. Honouring elders and ancestors is a vital aspect of tribal life, where survival depends upon continuity. People turn to the older generation to keep in touch with their traditions. In Maori culture, children are often given to their grandparents to be raised in a traditional way.

But we live in a world that often disregards or rejects its recent history. Many Western women vow to do things differently from their own mothers, believing that they can do better. We often raise our children to have aspirations outside the home, rather than within it. Although becoming a mother is increasingly a life choice in the West, rather than an inevitability, there is often confusion about how to do the job well.

It's time now to take out the family photo album, to talk to our grandmothers – and our great-grandmothers, if we have them. We need to access our own matrilineal history, and take our place in the mother-line – for the sake of our daughters and our daughters' daughters.

Bibliography

Aria, Barbara *Mamatoto: A Celebration of Birth* (Virago Press, London, 1991)

Balaskas, Janet *Natural Pregnancy: A Practical, Holistic Guide to Wellbeing from Conception to Birth* (Gaia Books, London and Interlink Publishing Group, New York, 1990)

Blanks, Tim (ed.) *The Body Shop Book* (Little, Brown & Co., London, 1994)

Campion, Kitty *Holistic Herbal for Mother and Baby* (Bloomsbury Publishing, London, 1996)

Crystal, David *Listen to Your Child: A Parent's Guide to Children's Language* (Penguin Books, London and New York, 1986)

Culpeper, Nicholas *Culpeper's Book of Birth*, Ian Thomas (ed.) (Webb & Bower, Exeter, Devon, 1985)

Gavin, Jamila *Our Favourite Stories* (Dorling Kindersley, London and New York, 1997)

Goldin, Hyman E. *The Jewish Woman and her Home* (Hebrew Publishing Co., New York, 1941)

Hessing, Perle *A Mirror to My Life* (Cameron Books, London, 1987)

Hoffman, Mary and Ray, Jane *Song of the Earth* (Orion Books, London, 1995)

Husain, Shahrukh *The Goddess* (Macmillan, London and Little, Brown & Co., Boston, 1997)

Jackson, Adam J. *Eye Signs* (Thorsons, London, 1995)

Jackson, Deborah *Three in a Bed* (Bloomsbury Publishing, London, 1989)

Kindersley, Anabel and Barnabas *Children Just Like Me: Celebrations* (Dorling Kindersley, London and New York, 1995)

Kitzinger, Sheila *The Crying Baby* (Penguin Books, London and New York, 1990)

Kitzinger, Sheila (ed.) *The Midwife Challenge* (Pandora Press, Ontario, 1988)

La Leche League *The Womanly Art of Breastfeeding* (Penguin Books, London and New York, 1997)

Marks, Anthony and Tingay, Graham *The Romans* (Usborne Publishing, London and EDC Publications, San José 1990)

Milord, Susan *Hands Around the World: 365 Creative Ways to Encourage Cultural Awareness and Global Respect* (Williamson Publishing, Vermont, 1992)

Montagu, Ashley *Touching: The Human Significance of the Skin* (HarperCollins Publishers, London and New York, 1986)

Morris, Desmond *Babywatching* (Ebury Press, London, 1995)

Pilling, Ann, *Creation: Stories From Around the World* (Walker Books, London, 1997)

Priya, Jacqeline Vincent *Birth Traditions & Modern Pregnancy Care* (Element, Shaftesbury, Dorset, 1992)

Rose, Clare *Children's Clothes* (B.T. Batsford, London, 1989)

Rudd, Carol *Flower Essences* (Element, Shaftesbury, Dorset and Penguin, New York, 1998)

Stewart, R. J. *Celtic Gods, Celtic Goddesses* (Blandford Press, London, 1992)

Sutherland, Anne (ed.) *Face Values* (BBC Books, London, 1978)

Taylor, Colin *North American Indians* (Parragon Books, Bristol, 1997)

Willes, Margaret *Memories of Childhood* (The National Trust, London, 1997)

Index

Useful Addresses

United Kingdom

The Active Birth Centre
25 Bickerton Road
London
N19 5JT
Tel: 0171 482 5555

The Association of Radical
Midwives
62 Greetby Hill
Ormskirk
Lancashire
Tel: 01695 572776

Foresight
28 The Paddock
Godalming
Surrey
GU7 1XD
Tel: 01483 427839

La Leche League (GB)
BM 3424
London
WC1N 3XX
Tel: 0171 242 1278

USA and Canada

Billings Natural FP
316 North 7th Avenue
St Cloud
MN 56303
Tel: 1 888 867 6371

Doulas of North America
1100 23rd Avenue East
Seattle
WA 98112
Tel: 206 324 5440

La Leche League
International
1400 Meacham Road
Schaumburg
IL 60173
Tel: 847 519 7730

La Leche League of Canada
493 Main Street
Winchester
Ontario
KOC 2KO
Tel: 613 448 1842

Australia and New Zealand

Home Midwifery Association
(QLD) Inc.
PO Box 655
Spring Hill
Queensland 4000
Tel: 0732 551525

Homebirth Australia
PO Box 107
Lawson
NSW 2783
Tel: 0470 592014

La Leche League (NZ)
20 Douglas Avenue
Mount Albert
Auckland 3
Tel: 09 846 9612

Natural Family Planning
(NZ)
PO Box 5057
Whangarei
Tel: 09 438 8031